Gentle

NUTRITION

A Non-Diet Approach to Healthy Eating

RACHAEL HARTLEY, RD

Victory Belt Publishing Inc.

Las Vegas

First published in 2021 by Victory Belt Publishing Inc.

Copyright © 2021 Rachael Hartley

ISBN-13: 978-1-628604-24-5

Author photos by Holly Heaton

Cover design by Charisse Reyes

Interior design by Yordan Terziev and Boryana Yordanova

Printed in Canada
TC 0121

Contents

Introduction

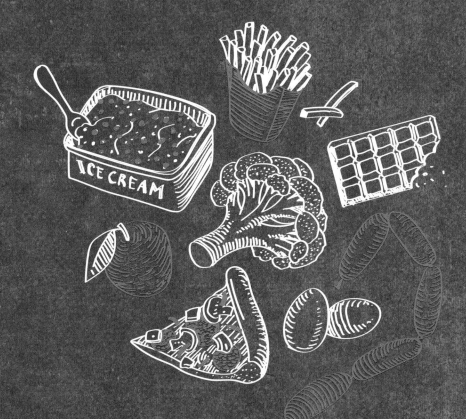

HOW WOULD YOU EAT IF YOU WEREN'T TRYING TO LOSE WEIGHT?

This is a question I come back to again and again with my clients. If you're like them, your first thought probably involves copious amounts of ice cream, pizza, and french fries. But I want you to sit on that question for a minute and, this time, *really* think about what your answer would be.

My guess is that it would still involve those foods because, well, they're pretty delicious. But I also think that there would be a limit on the amounts of ice cream, pizza, and fries you'd eat because when you knew you could have those foods whenever you wanted, they wouldn't seem quite so special anymore.

Also, because taste buds can get bored, you'd probably want a wide variety of other tasty foods, including fruits and vegetables. And you might even enjoy them. With weight loss being irrelevant to your food choices, you'd probably stress a lot less about food and have more headspace for other things. You'd eat when hungry, stop when satisfied, and move on with your life until hungry again.

You probably wouldn't emotionally eat very often either—at least not in the way we traditionally conceptualize it, like crying into a pint of ice cream. Since no food was off-limits, and since you knew you could have it whenever you wanted, you'd be more likely to deal with your emotions in other ways, like going for a walk or calling a friend. And if you did decide to soothe your stress with a batch of freshly baked cookies, it might actually make you feel better since you wouldn't be eating those cookies with a side of guilt.

Now, it's possible that you might think nutrition would get thrown out along with the intention to lose weight. However, what I think would happen is that you'd find it easier to make healthy choices when not distracted by calories or which foods are allowed and not allowed on your diet. Instead of trying to make sense of the cacophony of confusing and conflicting diet rules, you'd start listening to *your body*—the body that wants to feel good.

What does the kind of eating that I've just described feel like to you? Exciting? Intriguing? Joyful?

What about *freeing*? After all, this is freedom—*food freedom*. When you find freedom with food, it opens up space for you to find freedom in other areas of life also: freedom to be yourself; freedom to live a life unshackled from self-condemnation and judgment from diet culture; freedom from the various food rules created by people who know nothing about you, your body, or your needs; freedom from seeing nutrition as being punishing and stressful; freedom to tune in to the still voice of your body and nourish it in the way it wants—and *deserves*—to be nourished.

This freedom is very much possible. I know this because I see it every day in my practice. It is the kind of eating that feels peaceful, nourishing, and *gentle*.

What Is Gentle Nutrition?

Gentle nutrition is a flexible, non-diet, and evidence-based approach to healthy eating, one that centers on you and your unique individual needs. We live in a world where weight is misconceived as the be-all and end-all of health and where most nutrition advice is built upon that misconception. But when nutrition advice aims to shrink bodies, there's an inherent conflict with good nutrition—the kind of nutrition that can actually improve your health. That's because dieting is all about cutting things out, whereas good nutrition is about adding things in. And good nutrition is *gentle nutrition*.

Gentle nutrition is what nutrition looks like when we close our ears to the unscientific and fearmongering babble that makes food out to be the enemy and, instead, listen to our body telling us what makes it feel good. Gentle nutrition is what nutrition looks like when we stop obsessing over every meal and snack. Gentle nutrition encourages us to step back and look at the big pictures—both the big picture of our eating patterns over time as well as the big picture of our health and how nutrition is merely one of the many factors that influence it.

Gentle nutrition is how we approach nutrition within the practice of a non-diet approach that has been developed to help you build a healthier relationship with food and your body. That approach is called *intuitive eating.*

What Is Intuitive Eating?

Regardless of how much you know about intuitive eating, it's always helpful to ground yourself in the basics. If you already have some knowledge of and experience with the practice, I hope this book gives you a more nuanced understanding of intuitive eating as well as some new language to help you communicate it to others. If you are newer to the practice, I hope this introduction helps lay the groundwork for what you will learn in this book.

Intuitive eating is a non-diet approach to eating developed by dietitians Evelyn Tribole, MS, RDN, CEDRD-S, and Elyse Resch, MS, RDN, CEDRD-S, whose groundbreaking book, *Intuitive Eating,* outlines the ten principles of their approach. Since its publication in 1995, over a hundred studies demonstrating the physical and mental health benefits of intuitive eating have been published. Tribole and Resch have also developed a certification program for dietitians and other providers, producing certified intuitive eating counselors located all over the world.

The goal of intuitive eating is to help you foster a healthier relationship with your body and food. Rather than keeping you focused on weight, which is just an arbitrary number on the scale, or obsessed with what, when, or how much to eat, intuitive eating puts you in charge. It teaches you to get back in touch with your body's natural hunger and fullness cues; it helps you make decisions about food by listening to your body and replacing inaccurate, confusing, and conflicting diet rules with simple, accurate, and evidence-based information about food.

Intuitive eating might seem inaccessible—far off from how you have been eating. However, you may be encouraged to know that this is actually how we were born to eat. If you've been around babies or children and watched them eat, you might have noticed how their eating can vary from day to day and from meal to meal. A client once told me how terrified she would be when it seemed like her child wouldn't eat anything one day only to gobble down their meals and snacks, asking for seconds, the next. Babies' eating typically balances itself out over time. It's when rules and restrictions around food are introduced that we begin to lose touch with the inner intuitive eater we were born to be.

Often, those first food rules are taught by well-meaning parents who want to instill healthy eating habits in their children. Told to eat our vegetables before getting dessert as a reward, we've been learning since early childhood that some foods are chores and some are treats. Told to clean our plates but not to eat too much dessert, the intuitive eater inside us is confused by these conflicting messages. Later—not that much later for some children, sadly—more food rules and restrictions are introduced through diet culture and its overwhelming fear of fatness. However, no matter how long you have been dieting, know that you have everything you need for a more peaceful and intuitive relationship with food.

Why Intuitive Eating?

Why intuitive eating? In short, because diets don't work.

Since you picked up this book, I'm guessing that you're already aware of this fact or at least are starting to come to grips with it. Most of my clients come to me feeling sick and tired of dieting. They've spent unbelievable amounts of time, energy, and money on all the things that they thought would help them lose weight and keep it off: counting calories (or points or macros), low-carb diets, Paleo diets, keto diets, clean eating, meal replacements, expensive gym memberships, support groups, fasting, detoxes, and often weird and clearly

The Ten Principles of Intuitive Eating

1. REJECT THE DIET MENTALITY

Rejecting the diet mentality is about rejecting the idea of diets altogether. It's about letting yourself get angry at diet culture along with its lies and false promises of permanent weight loss. It's about letting go of the hope that there's another diet out there that will "work." It's about chipping away at the belief that smaller is better or that weight is a marker of health, success, value, and worth.

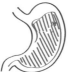

2. HONOR YOUR HUNGER

Instead of having your goal be to eat as little as possible, eat adequately throughout the day as a way of reframing your approach to food. Eating enough is the most important aspect of nutrition; it also prevents the primal hunger that triggers overeating and impulsive food choices. Learn to recognize hunger and to honor it.

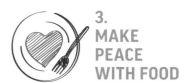

3. MAKE PEACE WITH FOOD

Making peace with food starts with giving yourself unconditional permission to eat all the foods you enjoy. Depriving yourself would only lead to intense cravings, frequent binges, and the kind of eating that feels out of control.

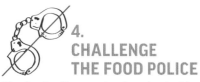

4. CHALLENGE THE FOOD POLICE

The food police are the thoughts inside your head that say you're being "good" or "bad" for eating a certain way. These unreasonable food rules create intense shame when you're not being "good." This shame can keep you trapped in the very behaviors that you're trying to change.

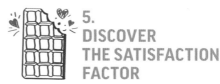

5. DISCOVER THE SATISFACTION FACTOR

Pleasure is an important aspect of healthy eating. The need to derive pleasure from food is literally built into the human DNA. Regardless of nutrition, everyone deserves to eat the foods they enjoy. Aiming for satisfaction enables you not only to determine when you've had "enough" but also to turn off those thoughts of food in order to allow headspace for other important and fun things in life.

unhealthy ways of eating—and yet a way of eating and exercising that leads to permanent weight loss still eludes them.

If this describes you, perhaps you've blamed yourself for being unable to stick to a diet plan. Or maybe you've wondered if your body is broken, as it stays the same size even when you *do* stick to a diet. I'm here to say that it's *not* you. The inability to lose weight permanently has almost nothing to do with willpower. What you see as your "failure" says a lot more about dieting than it does about you. In fact, despite the many "successful" weight loss stories you see glorified in magazines and on social media, only a very small number of people are able to lose weight and keep it off permanently. And many of these "successful" dieters engage in fairly obsessive and unhealthy behaviors in order to maintain that weight loss, which makes them arguably less healthy than they were before they embarked on a life of dieting.

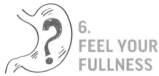

6. FEEL YOUR FULLNESS

Learn what it feels like to be satisfied but not stuffed. Fullness is not an uncomfortable sensation; it's not about eating only until hunger is no longer present either. Slowing down and checking in with your body can help you discover what it feels like to be comfortably full.

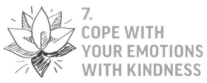

7. COPE WITH YOUR EMOTIONS WITH KINDNESS

Treat yourself kindly by building up a toolbox of skills to help cope with emotions, such as anxiety, boredom, sadness, and frustration, that might normally cause you to turn to food.

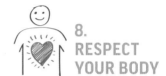

8. RESPECT YOUR BODY

Just as we have different heights, shoe sizes, and hair colors, we have different body sizes. And some of those sizes are large, above what BMI charts and mainstream beauty standards consider "ideal." These cultural standards are wrong, not the larger bodies. However, loving your looks isn't a requisite for intuitive eating. Regardless of how you feel about your body size or shape, you can still treat it with respect.

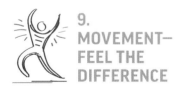

9. MOVEMENT— FEEL THE DIFFERENCE

Instead of moving your body with the goal of burning calories, focus on how it feels physically and mentally and engage in movement within your abilities that you enjoy.

10. HONOR YOUR HEALTH WITH GENTLE NUTRITION

Nutrition is part of health, not all of it. Take nutrition off its pedestal so you can engage with it in a gentle and flexible way. One meal or snack won't make or break your health. When you think about nutrition, think about the big picture rather than getting caught up in minutiae.

Adapted from *Intuitive Eating: A Revolutionary Program That Works,* by Evelyn Tribole and Elyse Resch

I want you to know that you're not alone. Every day in my practice, I meet people like you who live in a space that we in the intuitive eating community refer to as "diet rock bottom." They know from experience that diets don't work, but they feel lost without the rules and structure of a diet plan. Eating has always swung back and forth between all and nothing for them, and it's hard for them to imagine what that middle space even looks like.

This is where intuitive eating comes in. It is designed to get you out of that maddening dieting cycle. By putting intentional weight loss on the back burner, intuitive eating helps you learn how to tune in to your body's physical and emotional needs; it gives you permission to respond to those needs in whatever way you see fit. It helps you replace the confusing, conflicting, and stress-inducing diet rules with evidence-based nutrition information that enables you to nourish your body.

Essentially, intuitive eating helps you find that middle ground where you are able to self-moderate around food *and* allows you to give yourself a bit of compassion for the times you inevitably don't, since we're human beings who do human things, which sometimes include making mistakes with eating.

So, yes—if you want to boil it all down—I'm telling you to eat whatever you want, whenever you want. In fact, I'm telling you that eating this way might improve your health. Let's say goodbye to diet culture!

Health Benefits of Intuitive Eating

Although there is often a concern that healthy eating behaviors might go to the wayside when you take your focus off weight loss, not a single study has shown health risks associated with an intuitive eating approach. In fact, research has shown that intuitive eating and other non-diet approaches actually improve physiological markers, as well as health behaviors and psychological outcomes. The same can't be said for dieting and intentional weight loss.

A two-year study of an intuitive eating and size-acceptance intervention found improvements in blood pressure and cholesterol, as well as self-esteem, depression, and body image. A diet intervention, on the other hand, had resulted in some improvements to metabolic variables at the one-year mark, but those improvements were not sustained in year two. Furthermore, 41 percent of the participants dropped out of the diet group, whereas only 8 percent of those in the non-diet group did.[1]

A 2009 study found that intuitive eating and non-diet approaches improved health behaviors, including increased physical activity, increased consumption of fruits and vegetables, and decreased emotional eating and binge eating.[2]

A 2015 review of research into non-diet approaches found that not a single study showed a worsening of blood glucose, blood pressure, or cholesterol with the adoption of a non-diet approach.[3]

A review of twenty intuitive eating interventions found that intuitive eating reduced anxiety and depression as well as disordered eating behaviors, like binge eating and dietary restriction, while increasing quality of life.[4]

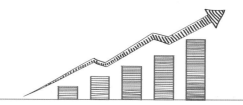

A Pursuit of Thinness or a Pursuit of Health?

Weight is a major part of how we conceptualize health. We've all been subjected to decades of the "obesity epidemic" rhetoric that has created an intense fear of being or becoming a higher weight. In your doctor's office, for example, you're far more likely to see a poster showing the BMI chart than one advocating health-promoting behaviors, like engaging in physical activity, getting adequate sleep, or not smoking. We are essentially told that being fat is a death sentence, so anxiety over food and body size seems warranted.

In reality, as Chapter 3 will discuss, weight plays a much smaller role in health than what we are told. Body diversity is real; just as some people are naturally thin, others are naturally large. A larger body size does not automatically indicate a health concern. With the exception of statistical extremes, both high *and* low, BMI only weakly predicts longevity.[5] In fact, for people over fifty-five years of age, having a BMI in the "overweight" or "obese" range is associated with a lower risk of death.[6] But that's probably not the message you're getting from your doctor, is it?

Pursuing health and wellness seems innocent enough. Who out there doesn't want to live a long and relatively illness-free life? Unfortunately, diet culture and its rigid rules for weight loss have become so inextricably wrapped up in nutrition that when someone gives you advice on healthy eating, it can be hard to know whether there is a whispered subtext of "and this might help you get thinner!" in there somewhere. Even when the goal is truly wellness and not weight control, diet culture still forces upon us rigid views of what qualifies as healthy eating.

And just as diets make you believe that you'll instantly gain weight from eating even slightly outside your plan, nutrition that has been influenced by diet culture makes you feel you've caused irreparable damage to your health when you take just one wrong bite of food. A cookie stops being a fun treat and becomes an inflammatory sugar bomb. A frozen meal stops being a convenient option for when you forget to pack lunch and becomes a stew of toxic additives. And fast food? Forget it!

Diet culture takes rational nutrition advice and blows it up to where it's no longer accurate or helpful. Clean eating is a perfect example. It started out as a push to eat more whole foods and fewer processed foods—nutrition advice that is perfectly reasonable. Over time, however, it has warped into a mess of silly food rules that are impossible to follow unless you have the time and money to cook everything from scratch using nothing but organic ingredients. The rise in popularity of clean eating has led to an increase in a type of disordered eating called orthorexia, an unhealthy obsession with eating in a way one considers to be healthy, which can cause the same physical and psychological side effects that anorexia does.

When nutrition is rigid and restrictive, it becomes unsustainable and unhealthy. No amount of green juice or organic berries can make up for the missing nutrients from cutting out food groups or for the stress on the body from obsessing and stressing about food. In contrast, intuitive eating offers a gentle, flexible approach to healthy eating—one that truly honors both physical and mental health.

How Intuitive Eating Changed My Practice

When I first started practicing as a dietitian over a decade ago, I practiced in a very traditional sense. I taught my clients calorie counting, portion control, and all the tips and tricks I thought would help them lose weight and keep it off for good. My approach to health and nutrition was very much influenced by the clean eating movement that was ramping up at the time.

In my mind, I was a sensible dietitian because I believed that all foods fit—even if you had to do some calorie counting or restricting later on to make room for them. I wasn't promoting fad diets or quick fixes for weight loss; I believed in making what I thought were small, sustainable changes. Surely I wasn't doing anything irresponsible to promote unhealthy relationships with food, right?

Wrong.

After working as an inpatient, hospital-based dietitian for a couple of years, I moved into a role as an outpatient dietitian at a large medical center, where I began to see clients who had been referred to me by their doctors for medical concerns, like diabetes or high cholesterol, and for weight loss. As a relatively new dietitian, I found this to be a dream job. I looked forward to moving from seeing clients just once or twice while they were in the hospital to being able to develop long-term relationships with them. I was thrilled at the prospect of helping my clients make sustainable, health-promoting changes and develop their own sets of before-and-after pictures.

But that didn't materialize the way I'd hoped. What happened was that my clients would initially lose weight only to gain it back quickly. Their eating patterns became chaotic, swinging back and forth between following my advice with extreme rigidity and bingeing on or overeating the foods that I had told them to limit. Or they would make lots of healthy changes to their eating habits, but the scale wouldn't budge. Soon, frustrated with the lack of progress despite eating healthier, they would go back to the way they'd been eating before.

I couldn't understand what was going on. I felt confident in my interactions. After all, on a patient satisfaction survey, my services were ranked as excellent. Why weren't my outcomes just as good? Just as my clients were feeling like a failure, I was feeling like a professional failure. I started to second-guess my career choice, convinced that there was something wrong with me that made me a bad dietitian.

When I discovered intuitive eating, everything fell into place for me. I came to recognize how restriction leads to bingeing and overeating, which explains the chaotic eating patterns I was witnessing among my clients. I came to understand how calorie restriction slows your metabolism, which explains why someone could eat less and not lose weight. I came to see the psychological effects of dieting and how demonizing foods as "off-limits" only puts those foods up on a pedestal, inevitably resulting in "Last Supper eating" where you eat something off your diet plan as if you were eating your last supper, telling yourself that you'll go back to your diet on Monday. I dug into weight science and learned how weight and health are not one and the same and how body diversity naturally exists. I learned how the cultural obsession with thinness stems from a fear of fatness that's based on harmful and inaccurate stereotypes and how these beliefs directly contribute to the inhumane treatment of larger-bodied individuals, especially in healthcare systems. I saw how the focus on weight promotes unhealthy relationships with food, including eating disorders and disordered eating, both of which are much more prevalent than I was taught in school. Finally, I came to understand that the problem is neither me nor my clients but the entire system of dieting and the weight-centric health paradigm.

My practice didn't change overnight. Just as someone's personal journey to peace with food is a lifelong affair, so too is my professional journey of unlearning decades of misinformation about food, weight, and health and relearning how to practice in a way that honors all bodies and lived experiences. But, in having ditched diets professionally and having brought intuitive eating into my practice, I came to see the power of this work. My clients have learned to build a healthier relationship with food; they have broken out of their unwanted food habits and fostered new and healthier ones that are rooted in self-care as opposed to self-deprivation. I don't have an album of my clients' before-and-after pictures—I'd been taught that was the goal—but I have witnessed their before-and-after lives, something so much more valuable to them and to me.

The Goal of This Book

My goal in writing this book, first and foremost, is to provide a non-diet resource on nutrition and to demonstrate what nutrition looks like when we remove the assumption that weight equals health.

As a resource on nutrition, *Gentle Nutrition* helps you combat the fearmongering about nutrition and health that can be a major barrier to healing your relationship with food. Social media, for example, is where nutrition myths and misconceptions can flourish. Anyone can pose as a nutrition expert, as long as they are thin and fit. With this book, I want to help you unlearn those falsehoods and replace them with flexible, evidence-based nutrition knowledge.

As an exploration of the role of nutrition in the context of intuitive eating, *Gentle Nutrition* serves as a resource for those who want to engage with nutrition outside diet culture. It aims to make non-diet information about food and nutrition accessible to more people. While having the intention to eat healthier is by no means an obligation, it is a concern for many and a priority for some. I believe that *you* get to decide how you want to feed your body and whether nutrition is going to factor into that decision. And if it is, you deserve access to good information. Having a better understanding of nutrition science will also help you make peace with food through an understanding of how the body uses different foods and nutrients.

This book also seeks to debunk the unfortunate myth that intuitive eating is anti-nutrition. This stems from the fact that nutrition is often conceptualized through restriction, deprivation, and dieting. When people talk about getting healthy, it can be assumed that they mean losing weight. So, with intuitive eating telling you to ditch dieting, it's easy to see why it's viewed as anti-nutrition. But this couldn't be further from the truth. Nutrition is immensely important in intuitive eating; gentle nutrition is one of the ten principles of intuitive eating, after all.

I believe in the power of good nutrition to improve people's lives. Otherwise, I wouldn't have dedicated six years of my life to studying nutrition and twelve years to practicing it. At first, I believed good nutrition meant weight control and "clean" eating. However, through self-reflection and an honest appraisal of my practice, I came to see that what I was doing wasn't actually helping people eat any better, let alone live a happier or healthier life. There are so many deeply ingrained assumptions and biases—so much misunderstanding and fear around weight and health—that have led most dietitians and healthcare providers to resort to nutrition approaches that hurt more than they help. Now that I've seen clearly the harm caused by the mainstream approach to nutrition and health that I was practicing, I can say with confidence that if I hadn't discovered intuitive eating, I would not be practicing as a dietitian today.

While this book focuses on the gentle nutrition aspect of intuitive eating, there are so many other incredible resources on intuitive eating out there, including books that dive into topics like the complexities of weight science, the history of diet culture, body image, and intuitive eating in eating disorder recovery. There is *so* much out there to learn for those who are interested. Since discovering intuitive eating and non-diet nutrition, the stack of books by my bedside has grown exponentially. If this book is your first introduction to intuitive eating, I hope that it whets your appetite to learn more.

In writing about something as personal as food, nutrition, and health, I think it's important to acknowledge my many privileges. As a thin, white, able-bodied, cisgender woman who has never struggled with food insecurity or received pressure from loved ones or healthcare providers to lose weight, I know that diet culture has not impacted me to the same degree that it has others. While I have listened to and learned from people whose experiences differ from mine, I am aware that there may still be blind spots in this book. I also recognize that non-diet messages from someone who has lived with these privileges may create a degree of resistance in some people. If that is the case, I hope you will explore the work of my fellow non-diet dietitians who are not thin, white women, such as Kimmie Singh, Amee Severson, Veronica Garnett, Christyna Johnson, Erica Leon, Glenys Oyston, and Aaron Flores, as well as body image experts like Sonya Renee Taylor, Briana Campos, Ashlee Bennett, Jes Baker, Shira Rose, and Meredith Noble, whose work has informed my practice.

Lastly, I have included in this book over fifty delicious new recipes for you to try. Those of you who have followed my blog know that I love cooking and getting creative in the kitchen. In creating these recipes, I tried to highlight a wide range of foods, including many common "fear foods," to show you that no foods are off-limits and that all foods can be incorporated into healthy eating patterns. Cooking can be a fantastic tool for strengthening your intuitive eating practice, and I hope that these recipes demonstrate how to incorporate nutrition in a fun and flexible way.

Above all, I hope that this book will make gentle nutrition seem more approachable to you. With diet culture making nutrition so rigid and restrictive as to be unsustainable, or manipulating the scale as a way of achieving health, it has made good nutrition off-limits. It is my hope that this book brings nutrition back down to earth so that it's accessible to you again.

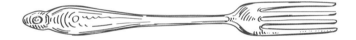

Part 1

THE
PRINCIPLES

Over the past year of writing, I've been asked countless times what my book is about by friends, relatives, and clients. It's been hard to find the words to succinctly summarize everything I wanted to include in this book, but I think I finally was able to home in on a simple thesis: if you want to eat healthier, you have to chill out about food a bit.

In my six years of studying nutrition and twelve years of practice as a dietitian, I've learned a lot about the science of nutrition, health, and food. In school, I pulled all-nighters to memorize diagrams of the metabolic pathways that turn macronutrients into energy and the vitamin and mineral content of various foods and to understand the research on various therapeutic diets for specific health conditions. As I've settled into my career, however, I've come to appreciate the fact that despite the complexities of nutrition science, what you need to know to feed your body well is actually quite simple.

Unfortunately, most of the popular discourse about nutrition doesn't make it appear that way. Some foods go—seemingly overnight—from being demonized to being given superfood status and vice versa. The diets that are in vogue become ever more complex. Famous nutrition gurus and wellness influencers share confusing and conflicting messages along with cherry-picked science to prove that their way is the "right" way.

Besides, nutrition has become inextricably tied to our cultural anxieties about weight. Popular nutrition advice is rarely *truly* about health but rather how to shrink your body, albeit temporarily. With all the pressure around food, it's no wonder so many people feel anxious about every meal or snack, wondering if what they are eating is "right" or "wrong."

In this book, I will discuss how this anxiety about food and weight is actually making you less healthy, as it adds unnecessary stress to your life and keeps you trapped in chaotic cycles of food deprivation, followed by bingeing and backlash eating. I will introduce a non-diet approach to nutrition called *intuitive eating,* which is a way to reprogram your thinking, removing diet culture's most insidious messaging from it and replacing it with a more flexible and evidence-based approach to nutrition called *gentle nutrition.*

Chapter 1

WHY DIETS
DON'T WORK

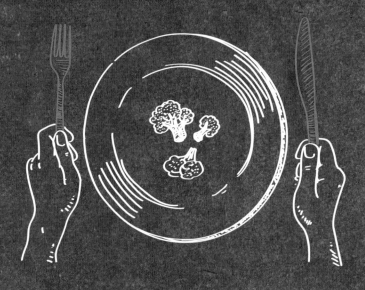

If there is one message that needs to come through loud and clear in this chapter and in this book, it's that it's not your fault that the million diets you've tried have failed.

I can't tell you how many conversations I've had with clients in which they express that their lack of success at dieting is due to personal faults and that they feel like a failure. I can't tell you how many of them have said to me that they're lazy or they have no willpower. These are the same people who have accomplished things like starting their own business, raising children while taking care of a sick loved one, or completing an intense postgraduate program while holding a job on the side.

One reason I spend so much time talking with my clients about why dieting doesn't work is that I consider it one of my primary responsibilities as a dietitian to alleviate the shame they feel about their eating behaviors and their bodies. Shame harms physical and mental health and keeps us trapped in destructive disordered eating behaviors. How can you break free from the dieting cycle or treat your body with care if you believe that you are somehow defective?

With dieting, we set unreasonable standards, and then we try to bully ourselves into submission with cruel self-talk. Would you talk to someone else the way you talk to yourself? Would you tell a friend they are hopeless because they couldn't stay away from the chips and dip at a work event? Would you call a friend lazy for sleeping in past a 6 a.m. workout? Would you think there was something wrong with them for not being able to stick to their low-calorie meal plan? I'd hope not!

Most of us recognize that shaming someone else isn't helpful, yet we continue to shame ourselves with negative self-talk and somehow expect it to motivate change.

Now, I'm not saying this so you can try to positive self-talk your way into sticking to a diet plan. Nope, this is not a "love yourself thin" diet book! The problem is that the diet itself is an unreasonable standard, and it sets you up for failure. Instead of thinking you are the problem, let's look at *diets* as the problem.

Why Diets Aren't the Answer

Diets have become harder to spot these days, with the diet industry starting to rebrand their plans, books, and products as "wellness" after realizing that the diet brand is going out of fashion. And since the weight loss aspect of it is no longer explicit but subtly implied, diets have become harder to spot these days, and things have become very confusing.

Therefore, let me state that, for the purpose of this book, I consider a diet to be any eating plan or any set of guidelines that promises or implies weight loss as an outcome, and I consider someone to be dieting whenever they engage in behavior changes of any kind with an expectation of weight loss.

However, I want to make a distinction between that type of diets and the kind of medical diets that are prescribed appropriately, like a gluten-free diet for people with celiac disease. The word "diet" in the latter case carries a completely different meaning. It's also important to note that the word is also often used to describe dietary patterns, as in the standard American diet or the Mediterranean diet, or to describe an individual's eating patterns. In this case, it's used as a descriptor and doesn't necessarily connote weight loss.

Diets Don't Work!

- One study examined over 175,000 men and women with BMIs greater than 30, who were enrolled in weight loss studies, and found a 0.004 percent chance for men and a 0.01 percent chance for women of attaining a "normal" BMI between 20 and 25. For those with a BMI between 40 and 45, the probability dropped to 0.0008 percent for men and 0.001 percent for women.[7]

- What about that reasonable 5 percent weight loss you always hear about? That's a 10-pound loss for a 200-pound person. The same study found a one in eight chance of maintaining that weight loss for nine years for men and a one in seven chance for women.

- A 2009 review examining forty-seven workplace wellness programs found that, after three to six months, those who participated in the programs lost an average of only 3 pounds more than those who did not participate.[8]

- Not only do diets not work, they may also contribute to weight gain over time. Studies show that one-third to two-thirds of dieters regain more weight than they lost on their diets.[9] There's nothing wrong with gaining weight, but that's obviously not the outcome people are hoping for when they start a diet.

- A 2019 review of weight loss studies with at least three years of follow-up found that the average rate of weight regain is 0.14 percent each month, which means that the average participant will reach their pre-intervention weight after about four years. This is consistent with other studies showing that most people regain the weight within about five years.[10]

- For all the headlines you see touting the benefits of various diets and success stories, there is not a single study showing that permanent weight loss is possible for more than a small percentage of people.

Let's now turn our attention to some research findings that show us why diets don't work—at least not in the long term. While short-term weight loss can be achieved through a variety of methods, research shows that maintaining weight loss is much more challenging. In 2013, a group of researchers examined every single randomized controlled trial of weight loss interventions that included a follow-up of at least two years (a total of twenty-one studies—a surprisingly low number given the assumption of most researchers and healthcare professionals that anyone can lose weight and keep it off). Through the study, the researchers found that the dieters lost weight in the first year only to gain back all but an average of 2.1 pounds over the next two to five years.[11]

All that headspace, time, money, and effort for 2.1 pounds? I don't think I've met anyone who embarks on a diet with a goal of losing 2.1 pounds or to lose weight and gain it all back. This research on thousands of individuals shows that if your attempts to lose weight have ended in failure, you are not alone. It also shows that for all of mainstream healthcare's focus on achieving a "healthy" BMI, it hasn't found a way for more than a small number of people to do so.

Why is it so hard to keep the weight off? Well, it all goes back to how human beings evolved. Historically, starvation has been the greatest threat to our survival, and because of that, we have evolved different mechanisms to protect against it. While our environment has changed significantly since those early hunter-gatherer days, our brain has remained mostly the same. So, even though you may feel frustrated as you learn about the biological mechanisms that fight against weight loss, remember that they are there for a purpose. Your body is just doing its best to keep you alive. A diet not working is actually a beautiful sign of our body working the way it's supposed to, although it's hard to see it as such against the backdrop of our fatphobic culture.

Due to these mechanisms, as you take in fewer calories than your body uses each day in an attempt to lose weight, your body interprets the energy deficit as a threat to survival, namely starvation. Your body doesn't know you're trying to lose weight; it doesn't know you're not eating carbs because it's bathing suit season. As far as your body is concerned, not eating enough has historically meant only one thing, and that is no access to enough food.

To illustrate how the body protects against starvation, I want you to imagine a hungry caveperson ancestor of yours. Let's pretend they have gone days between mastodon hunts, or they can't find any safe plants to eat. What do you think their brain would have their body do to keep them alive? It might send out hunger cues and thoughts about food so that the caveperson becomes highly motivated to seek out something to eat. It also might tell their body to slow down energy use so as not to waste energy on nonessential activities like reproduction (hence the low sex drive and wonky hormones when dieting). It also might send out signals making energy-dense foods seem extra palatable so your ancestor isn't wasting their time foraging for plants when what they really need is a nice piece of juicy, fatty meat.

These protective mechanisms are best illustrated with an analogy shared by neuroscientist Sandra Aamodt in her 2013 TED Talk on why diets don't work.[12] She compares the brain to a thermostat that's been set to keep our body weight within a natural set-point range. The thermostat's job is to keep your house at the temperature at which it's set, regardless of the weather. You could open a window in the winter to try to lower the temperature, but the thermostat is just going to kick in, and the heating system will work even harder to bring your house to the set temperature. You could try to fight it by keeping all your doors and windows open all winter, but you would likely break your heating system. It's the same with dieting. The more you try to overpower the system, the harder it will work against your efforts. In order to keep your body weight within your natural set-point range, your brain has to adjust things, like hunger, activity levels, and metabolism. You could continually try to override your body's natural set point, but you would likely cause it to break down. When the stated purpose of pursuing weight loss is to improve health, does it really make sense to put your body through something that literally forces it to fight for survival?

The Biological Adaptations to Dieting

One of the ways our body adapts to restriction is with hunger and fullness hormones. Hunger and fullness cues are regulated by a variety of hormones, chief among which are ghrelin and leptin. Among other functions, ghrelin works as the "hunger hormone," which naturally increases before a meal and lowers as one eats enough food to fuel one's body. Leptin is almost the opposite of ghrelin; it functions as the "satiety hormone" that inhibits hunger. When you're adequately nourished, the hypothalamus, the part of your brain that acts like a hormone command center, controls the release of ghrelin and leptin to regulate intake according to your energy needs. It accommodates for the times you need more energy, like after an intense activity, and the times you need less energy.

However, when you're undernourished, ghrelin levels stay elevated, even after eating a normal-sized meal.[13] In fact, studies have found that ghrelin levels remain elevated and leptin levels reduced for as long as a year after weight loss.[14] At the same time, metabolism, the body's energy expenditure, drops with weight loss. Most of us probably recognize this on a logical level: a smaller body generally requires less fuel than a larger body. This is because there's less body mass to pump blood through, move around, and keep at 98.6°F. However, when this smaller body is achieved through dieting and restriction, metabolism will drop more than expected. One of the most widely known examples of this is the "*Biggest Loser* Study," where sixteen participants of the popular (and incredibly cruel) weight loss show had their metabolism and body composition measured at the end of the competition, and then again six years later. They found that the participants needed about 500 fewer calories per day than expected for someone of a similar height, weight, and age. The winner of that season needed a whopping 800 fewer calories than expected.[15] This caloric adaptation was found regardless of whether the participants maintained most of the weight loss or gained it back, and almost all the contestants gained the weight back.

Obviously, *The Biggest Loser* is a pretty extreme example—with its participants following an extremely rigid diet plan while exercising close to ten hours a day, literally turning dieting into their full-time job! And even though other studies don't show that extreme level of metabolic adaptation, it's still significant, especially if you factor in the increase in hunger. To put it in perspective, for every kilogram (2.2 pounds) of weight lost, appetite increases by a hundred calories per day, while metabolism drops by twenty to thirty calories per day.[16]

There have been so many times that a client would sit across from me in my office, tearful and frustrated with the fact that the diet they've been sticking to is no longer working. They can't understand why one minor deviation results in multiple pounds gained. Sometimes their friends or family don't believe that they actually eat what or how much they say they eat; sometimes those friends and family make comments implying that they must be cheating on their diet. If that's you, know that I believe you. Having spent so much of their life fighting biology, the chronic dieters I work with have some of the strongest willpower I've ever seen.

The Psychological Effects of Dieting

It's not only your biology that fights against your attempts to lose weight, but your psychology as well. If you find yourself thinking about food constantly while on a diet, it's not because you're a food-crazed eating machine. This has little to do with your willpower and a lot to do with the impact that dieting has on the brain. What happens here is that you're dealing with a pretty typical side effect of dieting—food obsessions. This makes sense when you realize that thinking about food is a common sign of hunger!

To normalize food obsessions and help my clients understand what they're experiencing, I like to tell them about Ancel Keys' Minnesota Starvation Study.[17] The goal of the study was to better understand the impact of malnutrition and to learn how to refeed safely. Although not the most ethical study, it tells us a lot about the physical and psychological effects of calorie deprivation. The study was conducted toward the end of World War II as the Allied forces were making their way through German-occupied Europe, encountering civilians, who had little access to food apart from bread and potatoes, as well as survivors at concentration camps, who had suffered even more extreme starvation and malnutrition. Keys recruited thirty-six healthy young men, who were conscientious objectors of war, and subjected them to semi-starvation. During the study, the participants were fed a diet that was nutritionally designed to replicate the diet of war-torn Europe, which consisted of mostly root vegetables and bread, supplemented with a bit of butter, oil, and dairy.

One thing that the researchers found surprising was that besides the physical side effects of dizziness, fatigue, hair loss, anemia, and muscle loss, the participants also developed extreme psychological side effects. They became anxious and depressed and had difficulty concentrating. Two participants even required brief hospitalizations in the acute psychiatric ward. One of the most significant effects that the researchers noticed was the men's intense preoccupation with food. These men lost interest in all other subjects and activities and began reading cookbooks and trading and collecting recipes; sometimes they stayed up until the early morning hours, engaging in these food-related activities. Some of the participants were so distracted by daydreams of food that they had to drop out of classes. One anecdote, recounted by a journalist who reported on the study, is about a participant who walked by a bakery and, tempted by the wafting scent of doughnuts, went inside, bought a dozen, and gave them to children just so he could watch them eat.

Even when the participants were refed and their weight restored at the end of the study, the food obsessions persisted for some time. One participant described his cravings as a hole that couldn't be satisfied by filling up his stomach. Even well after the study was over, a significant number of the men went on to have careers that involved food. Remember—these are twenty-year-old dudes in the 1940s, well before today's "foodie" culture!

I can almost hear you on the other end, "Well, they were *starving*! Of course, they would react like that! I have a much more sensible plan to follow!" Well, what if I told you that during the three-month-long period of semi-starvation, the participants were provided approximately 1,800 calories a day. That sounds like a feast compared to some of the diets I've seen in women's magazines!

You see, whenever you are taking in less energy and fewer macronutrients than your body needs, it has an effect on your brain that triggers intense food cravings. And while the Minnesota Starvation Study provides a particularly dramatic example, pretty much anyone who has been on a diet knows firsthand how restriction causes food obsessions. No matter how seemingly healthy or balanced an approach to weight loss may seem, it always involves restriction or deprivation of some kind. Otherwise, you would just eat what you want when you want. When you're deprived of something you want or need, you're going to crave it. Add to that the increased hunger cues we talked about before, and it's no wonder all those diets have failed!

This is where I repeat that chronic dieters have some of the strongest willpower of anyone I know. If this resonates with you, you know exactly what I'm talking about. You're literally living your life hanging by a thread trying to stick to your diet plan until something goes wrong and cuts it! With daydreams of food running through your head, a low blood sugar level, and fatigue, you can go into a tailspin just from one minor thing—something you'd have the headspace to deal with in a more helpful way when adequately nourished.

And when you give in—and that's inevitable—the eating that follows would probably feel pretty out of control. Remember the "Last Supper eating" mentioned earlier? That's likely what's going to happen. Who knows when you'll get to eat that forbidden food again, right? So, you better get it all in now! Also, there's often what I like to call the "eff it effect" where you tell yourself that since you've already blown your diet, well, *eff it*, you might as well just keep eating.

You could be thinking right now that you would still overeat those "bad" foods even if you weren't dieting. This may be partially true. Yes, all of us overeat from time to time, and that's fine! Sometimes we miss the mark; sometimes food is so enjoyable that we eat more of it than what feels good. But I promise: the vast majority of your eating experiences with forbidden foods will feel very different when your body is well nourished and when those foods are no longer off-limits. The common dieting trope of hunger being the best seasoning is literally true here. When you are calorie-deprived, foods, especially energy-dense foods, actually taste and smell better to you. On the other hand, when you are adequately nourished, and when you know that you can have any foods you like whenever you want, those forbidden foods are taken off the pedestal. At that point, you may still find those foods enjoyable or come to realize that you actually don't like them very much! Several clients have told me that they're finding the foods that they used to love and felt like they had no self-control around to be just so-so now that they've spent some time working on intuitive eating.

To sum up, restriction creates a situation where you're trying to eat less while your body is telling you to eat more and attempting to conserve the little bit of food you give it. The biological and psychological deprivation created by dieting leads to intense food cravings and obsessions, making it even harder to stick to your plan. If you feel burdened by a history of failed attempts at dieting, I hope this section takes some shame and blame off your shoulders.

The Dieting Cycle

I'm going to take a wild guess and say you're probably one of the vast majority of dieters whose attempts at weight loss didn't exactly go to plan. Otherwise, you probably would have put this book down after the first few pages.

Despite that, you may be looking back—with rose-colored glasses on—over the diets you've done in the past that have "worked," albeit temporarily, convincing yourself that it was your lack of willpower that did you in. You may still feel like there's another diet out there that just might work for you. Or perhaps you're intrigued by the idea of intuitive eating; you just want to come back to it after you've lost the weight first.

I think now is a good time to note that it's fine if you still want to lose weight. A common misconception about intuitive eating is that you cannot want to lose weight. This is simply untrue and unsympathetic to the immense pressures on people, *especially* larger-bodied people, to be thinner (also, if you didn't desire weight loss at all, you'd probably already be a pretty intuitive eater!). The culture we live in doesn't treat all body sizes equally. There are very real social advantages to having a thin body or one that's "curvy in the right places" for feminine-gendered people and to having a strong, muscular body for masculine-gendered people. People in larger bodies are treated horribly in our society, especially by the medical community that claims to be so concerned about their health. Fat bias in our society is very real and, sadly, often thought of as justified, as most people believe body size is something that is entirely within our control. Putting weight loss on the back burner is much easier said than done when you're experiencing marginalization for your body's shape or size (not to mention race, gender, sexual orientation, or disability). Because of this, I understand how difficult it can be to let go of trying to control your weight, and I could never blame anyone for wanting to lose weight or for actively trying to do so.

However, intuitive eating exists to provide you with an option to not spend your life fighting your body or being trapped in the dieting cycle. It gives you a set of tools to turn to when you want to take care of your body without trying to manipulate its size. I hope that the discussion on why diets don't work does not make you feel guilty if you're not ready or able to give up your desire for weight loss entirely. As you embark on this intuitive eating journey, a part of you may still want to lose weight; that's fine. Intuitive eating will teach you to deprioritize that desire and to keep it from influencing how you take care of your body. It will teach you to treat your body as if you were okay with it—even if that's not always how you feel. Because as much as you've been told that a smaller body is a prerequisite for health, as I will discuss further in Chapter 3, it's simply untrue. Regardless of your weight, size, or shape, you deserve to have a more peaceful relationship with food and your body and to have the freedom to engage with nutrition from a place of self-care, not punishment! You deserve to live your life free from the dieting cycle.

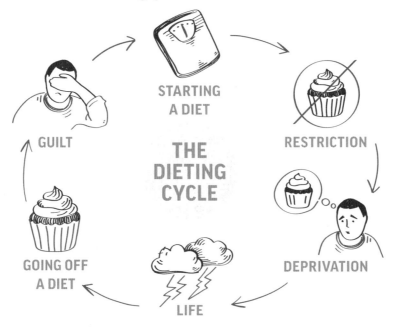

In the beginning of the dieting cycle, when you're just starting a new plan, things often feel really good, and the diet still feels relatively "easy" to follow at this point. You may be losing some weight; you could even experience a bit of a "dieter's high" where you're preoccupied with the expectation of weight loss and the excitement over how you think it will positively impact your life. But with time—it could be days, weeks, or months— deprivation builds and makes that diet harder to stick to. This is when you have to rely on immense amounts of willpower to stick to the plan.

Then something tough and unexpected pops up—it always does—and you find that the diet isn't flexible enough to accommodate for when life isn't smooth sailing. Think of all the time that goes into the planning, food prep, shopping, and workouts—not to mention the mental energy that goes into sticking to a diet. With your time and mental energy already in short supply when life gets stressful, you eventually slip. If you're like most of the chronic dieters I work with, that slip turns into the kind of eating that feels really out of control. This is not because you actually are out of control; it's all that built-up deprivation making you *feel* out of control.

I like to use a pendulum analogy to explain this to my clients. On one side of the pendulum is restriction and deprivation; on the other side, bingeing and overeating. Dieting pulls the pendulum all the way back toward restriction, and what happens when you let go? Eating swings back wildly toward bingeing and overeating.

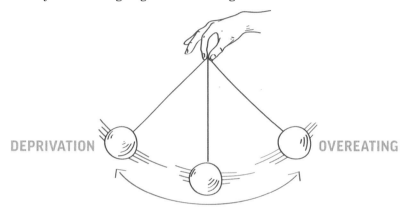

DEPRIVATION   OVEREATING

From the outside looking in, it's easy to see that the problem is the restriction; that's what causes the overeating and bingeing that feel so uncomfortable. But the dieter rarely sees it that way. After all, controlled, restrictive eating gets praised in our culture as discipline and taking care of one's health, whereas overeating is seen as laziness or a lack of self-control. Yet, instead of blaming the diet, the dieter blames themselves and feels immense guilt and shame for the perceived dietary indiscretions. In reality, what the dieter perceives as overeating may not even actually be overeating; often it's simply compensating or making up for the energy that their body hasn't been getting enough of!

However, overeating or bingeing is seen as the problem, whereas the restriction that fueled it isn't. Therefore, the way of dealing with the shame and the discomfort coming from these perceived dietary indiscretions is to go back on a diet. And the dieting cycle begins all over again.

Does this sound familiar to you?

Intuitive eating lets you take an off-ramp from this never-ending dieting cycle. Instead of trying to fix your body and to address your eating and health concerns with plans and restriction, intuitive eating gives you alternative ways of coping. Instead of pulling that pendulum back toward restriction yet again, you're now taking your hands off the pendulum and letting it settle in the middle. It's in this middle that there's space for gentle nutrition to come in and show you what it looks like to truly nourish your body.

Chapter 2
INTUITIVE
EATING

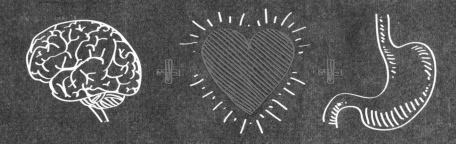

It's a frustrating paradox that eating, which is something we were born with the innate ability to do, has become as challenging and confusing as it is in our current diet culture. As human beings, we actually can manage eating well on our own; we got through the vast majority of our 200,000-year history without any knowledge of calories, nutrition, or diets.

But now it seems every food is wrong according to at least one authority figure. Bread, grains, pasta, and potatoes are too high in carbs. You can't eat beans because, supposedly, Paleolithic humans didn't eat them. Anything with more than five ingredients is out because it's clearly too processed. Gluten is out. Be careful with fat. Sugar consumption leads to every health condition imaginable. Nuts are healthy but have too many calories. And according to some of the newest diets, even vegetables aren't safe. Whew!

As you can see, even if you're not actively dieting, you're still dealing with so much noise about nutrition and what you should and shouldn't eat. And who could blame you for being so very, *very* confused and fearful? After all, some of the things you've read about food and nutrition are truly terrifying. Eating, which should be a simple, natural act, has consequently become stressful and overwhelming.

This is where intuitive eating comes in. This non-diet approach to eating helps you feed yourself without dieting, leads to a healthier relationship with food and your body, clears away the mess and confusion created by diet culture, and equips you with the knowledge of gentle nutrition so you can eat in a way that feels good for you without sacrificing the pleasure of eating and without obsessing about food all the time.

Who Is Intuitive Eating For?

Literally everyone.

Okay, so it's a bit more nuanced than that. But the simple answer is that since these principles are guidelines and *not* rules, they can be adapted to meet a wide range of needs. While some people may not be able to fully embrace intuitive eating, everyone can benefit from at least some aspects of it.

However, since its emphasis is on healing your relationship with food, intuitive eating often connects most strongly with people who identify as having struggled with an eating disorder or disordered eating. This group is actually larger than you might think. The most recent statistics on eating disorders reveal a lifetime prevalence of 8.4 percent for women and 2.2 percent for men.[18] And these numbers are likely to be low, as eating disorders are frequently missed, especially in higher-weight individuals, people of color, and those struggling with the kind of disordered eating that doesn't fit the diagnostic criteria. For example, one survey found that three out of four American women endorse unhealthy thoughts, feelings, or behaviors about food or their body. Dieting has become so normalized in our culture that not only are many of these behaviors not recognized as disordered, they're also often applauded as "healthy eating."

That said, some people may find certain aspects of intuitive eating more difficult to incorporate into their lives. These include people who lack food security, people who require a medical diet for a health condition, people who are diagnosed with a health condition that interferes with hunger and fullness cues, and people who have a history of trauma that makes tuning in to the body challenging. If these describe you, know that intuitive eating is still for you; you just have to focus on the aspects of it that may be more accessible to you.

Also, even though intuitive eating is commonly used in eating disorder recovery, some of its principles may not be appropriate early in treatment. For instance, someone who struggles with an eating disorder may not experience hunger, or they may feel fullness very quickly upon eating. In this case, the principle of using hunger and fullness cues to guide eating would not be as helpful to them as creating a meal plan to stabilize eating and to treat malnutrition. On the other hand, some principles, like making peace with food, would be vital to their healing.

Can I Lose Weight with Intuitive Eating?

New intuitive eaters often wonder if they will lose weight as a result. Certainly, it's possible to lose weight with intuitive eating. Others may gain or stay the same size. There's just no way to predict how your body will respond. Understandably, you may feel apprehensive about starting intuitive eating, not knowing how it will play out for you. No matter how intuitive eating affects your body size, it's not a reflection of whether you're doing it "right" or "wrong."

However, what I can tell you is that it will help your body settle in its set-point range, a weight range within which your body naturally fluctuates when it's fed adequately, well taken care of, and getting some amount of movement within its abilities. This is your healthy weight, not what the BMI scale says it should be.

I know that it's easier said than done, but please try to go into intuitive eating without expectations of weight loss. Better yet, trash your scale. It's not telling you anything important anyway. If giving up the scale entirely feels too scary, place it somewhere out of sight. Alternatively, set a journal on top of it so that the next time you're tempted to weigh yourself, you can journal what's going on. Often, in the course of journaling, you'll discover that what you're *really* looking for when you hop on the scale isn't something that's found in a number at all.

Four Themes of Intuitive Eating

There is so much information about the ten principles of intuitive eating that a book could easily be written on each of them. (If you'd like to take a deep dive into all the nuance of each principle, I highly recommend that you read the book *Intuitive Eating* by Evelyn Tribole and Elyse Resch, which I mentioned earlier.) For this reason, I've decided to keep the focus broad in order to cover more ground and to group these ten principles into four themes:

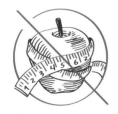
DITCHING DIETS

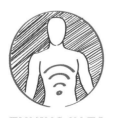
TUNING IN TO INTERNAL CUES

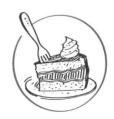
UNCONDITIONAL PERMISSION TO EAT ALL FOODS

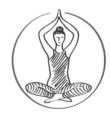
TREATING YOUR BODY KINDLY

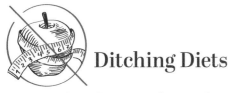

Ditching Diets

Ditching diets is much more than not being on a diet plan: in order to heal our relationship with food, we need to reject the *diet mentality* and put a stop to *pseudo-dieting*.

Diet mentality is a bit tricky to define, but essentially it is a mindset that values thinness and believes there is a right or wrong way or a right or wrong amount to eat.

Pseudo-dieting describes the ways in which the diet mentality influences our behaviors. Essentially, it's the more subtle ways of restricting food, listening to the "should" in the back of your mind rather than your actual physical needs or wants. You might be ordering a salad or skipping dessert or replacing potatoes with cauliflower not because you're on a diet, but rather out of a vague notion that the alternative is "bad." That's the diet mentality sneaking into your way of thinking and causing you to engage in pseudo-dieting behaviors that, as demonstrated in the pendulum analogy in Chapter 1, trigger backlash eating in the same way dieting does.

INTUITIVE EATING PRINCIPLES:

REJECT THE DIET MENTALITY.

RESPECT YOUR BODY.

Is Your Healthy Lifestyle a Diet in Disguise?

These days, diets have become more insidious, going undercover as "wellness" or a "lifestyle." But just because something doesn't involve calorie counting doesn't mean it's not a diet.

Here are some questions to ask yourself to see if your healthy lifestyle is really a diet in disguise. If your answer to any of these questions is yes, you might be on a pseudo-diet.

1. Do you label food as good or bad?

2. Do you think of food in numerical units—grams, calories, etc.?

3. When you gain weight, do you take it as a sign that you're doing something wrong?

4. Do you celebrate weight loss?

5. Are all of the people who represent your healthy way of eating or your lifestyle thin?

6. If you knew that a lifestyle would make you happier and healthier but would also cause you to gain weight, would you still adopt it?

7. Do you feel shame or pride for eating certain foods?

8. When you close your eyes and imagine yourself after having adopted a new way of eating or lifestyle for an extended period of time, are you in a smaller body?

Adapted from the work of Virgie Tovar.[19]

In ditching diets, it's helpful to, first of all, explore your personal history with dieting and to examine whether it's something that has actually served you. What was life like for you when you were dieting? How did it fit within your life? Was there anything you had to give up? Did you lose weight? What caused you to go off the diet? What happened to your weight afterward? Did you notice that losing weight was more challenging with subsequent diets? When you're able to see that this is a road you've been down possibly many times before, you will find it a bit easier to convince yourself not to get on that same road again.

Some of you, however, may consider some of your past diet attempts "successful." I think it's important that we redefine "success" here. If you eventually regain the weight that was lost, has the diet actually succeeded in meeting its stated purpose? Also, consider the side effects of dieting, which may include suppressed metabolism, hormonal issues, intense food cravings and obsessions, fatigue, poor digestion, difficulty concentrating, anxiety, disconnection from hunger and fullness cues, binge eating, loss of muscle mass, and mood swings. A medicine with these side effects wouldn't get approved!

Of course, it's hard to ditch diets if you think your here-and-now body is unacceptable, or if you are afraid that your body will change for the worse if you stop trying to control it. Thankfully, you don't have to absolutely love your body in order to ditch the diet mentality; you simply need some level of *body respect.*

Hilary Kinavey, MS, LPC, and Dana Sturtevant, MS, RD, a therapist-dietitian team and the founders of Body Trust®, have developed more nuanced language to discuss the four stages of working toward a positive body image. "Stages" may be a misnomer, as it implies a constant forward progression. In reality, you may pass in and out of these different levels throughout life as your body changes and as life events impact your body image.

BODY RESPECT
Body respect is treating your body kindly, regardless of how you feel about it. You may not like your body very much, but you choose to care for it regardless. That includes not engaging in restrictive dieting behaviors or punishing exercise.

BODY ACCEPTANCE
Body acceptance is accepting your here-and-now body and believing in its inherent value regardless of its appearance or abilities.

BODY TRUST
Body trust is listening to what your body is telling you about its needs and responding accordingly. It's similar to the building of trust in a relationship; it may not come easily in the beginning, but it grows and deepens over time. Eventually, you will come to trust that your body cues accurately represent your body's needs.

BODY LOVE
Body love is an appreciation for all that your body is and all that it allows you to do. To use the same relationship analogy, it's the kind of love you feel in a long-term relationship. Perhaps looks are part of that love, but it goes deeper than that.

In ditching diets, examine what you were hoping to get from weight loss. Think about it—if no one noticed your weight loss and nothing in your life changed, would you still want to lose weight? I encourage you to examine if there are things you can pursue in your here-and-now body—things that make you feel more confident, seek out or deepen relationships, improve health, wear the clothes you like, and more.

Ditching dieting is a lot more complex and nuanced than getting rid of your weight loss program membership or deciding to eat carbs again. It's a lifelong process of identifying and challenging the thoughts and behaviors that are rooted in the diet mentality, and it's not easy. So, if you can't leave the pursuit of weight loss at home as you embark on the intuitive eating journey, at least pack it in the trunk so it's not doing any backseat driving!

Health at Every Size®

People pursue weight loss for many reasons other than appearance. We have been subjected to decades of the "obesity epidemic" rhetoric that has instilled a deep fear of being at a higher weight, often likening it to a death sentence. And this is why we focus on managing weight instead of engaging in health behaviors that are actually within our control. This fatphobia has harmed individuals all over the weight spectrum. In particular, it has caused extreme harm to higher-weight individuals whose healthcare providers label them "lazy" or "noncompliant," attribute symptoms of their treatable health conditions to weight, and even deny them necessary medical treatments.[20]

As I will discuss further in the next chapter, weight is not health. Health is not something that's totally within our control: healthy or not, everyone deserves access to stigma-free healthcare. Regardless of one's weight, engaging in healthy habits improves health—it's as simple as that. In fact, statistically, individuals with a BMI greater than 30 who engage in physical activity, drink alcohol in moderation, eat more than five servings of fruits or vegetables daily, and don't smoke have the exact same health markers as individuals with a BMI in what's deemed the "normal range," who engage in those same behaviors, and are healthier than those who don't.[21]

Though it's true that there are associations between markers of health, certain diagnoses, and weight—both high and low—the association is actually much less significant than we've been told. And much of it can be attributed to the health effects of weight stigma, weight cycling (i.e., yo-yoing), and behaviors that both harm one's health and may contribute to weight gain for some people.

According to the Association of Size Diversity and Health, a nonprofit organization that owns the trademark for Health at Every Size® (HAES), HAES is a weight-inclusive approach to healthcare that rejects the use of BMI, weight, or size as a proxy for health. It recognizes that the pursuit of health is not a moral imperative; it promotes access to health-promoting behaviors and stigma-free healthcare for people of all bodies; it says that one's health cannot be judged based on appearance and that everyone deserves resources to improve their health without focusing on weight loss.

The principles of HAES are as follows:

1. Weight Inclusivity—respect for all bodies and rejection of the idea that weight equals health

2. Health Enhancement—support of health-promoting behaviors, at an individual and population level, that improve well-being

3. Respectful Care—healthcare that's free from stigma and bias

4. Eating for Wellbeing—flexible, internally driven eating for hunger and fullness, nutrition needs, and pleasure (i.e., intuitive eating)

5. Life-Enhancing Movement—support of accessible and pleasurable physical activity

Research has shown that this approach is associated with improved physical and mental health markers, including lipids, blood pressure, body image, and self-esteem, as well as a higher engagement in health behaviors, like physical activity.[22]

Tuning in to Internal Cues

By going on a diet, you've put someone else in control of your body—someone who tells you what and how much to eat. To rely on advice and rules from books and online calorie calculators or celebrities and social media influencers is to say that these people know more about what your body needs than you do.

The truth is that you were born with everything you need to feed your body adequately. When it comes to feeding your body, hunger and fullness cues are your body's way of communicating to you when to start eating and when to stop eating. You can trust these cues in the same way that you would any other body cue, such as when you feel you need to urinate, to sleep, or to drink a glass of water.

Diet culture has trained us to ignore these cues because it sees calories as inherently bad and believes that the "right" way to eat is to consume as few of them as possible without keeling over. However, a calorie is simply energy, specifically the amount of energy required to raise the temperature of one kilogram of water by 1°C. When you reframe calories as energy, the idea of going out of our way to minimize food intake doesn't really make much sense now, does it?

Instead of counting calories, look to hunger and fullness cues for guidance on your energy needs. The hypothalamus, a part of the brain, is responsible for assessing the body's energy needs and for sending out hunger and fullness cues accordingly.[23] It's able to detect a drop in blood glucose and to send out hormones that trigger hunger. When you eat, the hypothalamus is able to detect a rise in blood glucose, amino acids, and fatty acids, along with the stretch of stomach muscles, and to respond by signaling fullness when you've had enough.

However, energy needs aren't static. The number of calories that your body needs changes from day to day and is affected by many things. Just remember that when it comes to meeting these changing needs, you don't need to hit a bull's-eye; you only need to get the dart on the board most of the time. And your hunger and fullness cues will guide you.

A perfect example of how humans can be flexible around food is the result of a 2006 study of twenty-six weight-stable individuals, which measured the amount of food these individuals ate each day and plotted it out over the course of a year. While the graph showed a wide variability in how much food they ate from day to day, their weight remained stable within their set-point range.[24]

Being able to listen to your hunger and fullness cues is great, but this can be a challenge when you have a long history of dieting, restricting, and bingeing. This is because dieting frequently asks you to ignore hunger, suppressing it until it reaches extreme levels that cannot be ignored. Then when you finally eat, the sense of panic and the need to get rid of the uncomfortable hunger drive you to blow past the point of fullness. Hunger and fullness, consequently, have become extreme sensations instead of the more comfortable levels in the middle where you're more likely to have the headspace you need to make a more intentional choice on how to feed yourself.

However, intuitive eating is not a hunger-fullness diet. You're not wrong for leaving a meal feeling overly full or wishing you ate more—sometimes we miss the mark. Also, there are many perfectly valid reasons to eat when you aren't physically hungry. There are three other types of hunger outside of physical hunger; all of them are perfectly valid reasons to eat.

Why You Should Delete Your Calorie Counting App

In general, online calorie calculators use either one of the two formulas for predicting basal metabolic rate (BMR): the Mifflin-St Jeor Equation and the Harris-Benedict Equation. These formulas are helpful in getting a ballpark estimate of BMR. However, these formulas aren't perfect. There are many aspects outside of anthropometrics that influence energy needs:

BODY COMPOSITION: Muscle tissue is highly metabolically active, so people who have more muscle have higher energy needs.

GENETICS: Genetics can influence one's energy needs.

GUT MICROBIOME: Gut bacteria play a role in extracting nutrients from food, and some are more efficient than others.

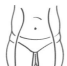

DIET HISTORY: People who have lost significant weight or have a history of restrictive dieting may have suppressed metabolism. This is commonly referred to as "starvation mode."

MEDICATIONS: Certain medications can increase or decrease metabolism.

MEDICAL HISTORY: Certain illnesses increase or decrease energy needs.

These factors are not accounted for in BMR formulas, which were developed in predominantly white research groups, whose weights were lower than average, and thus appear to be less accurate for people of color and for higher-weight individuals.[25]

Even if the formulas were accurate, the calorie counts on food aren't. Food companies are allowed to use any one of five different methods to calculate nutrition facts and to have a margin of error of up to 20 percent.[26] Calorie ranges for food were initially developed about 125 years ago by a scientist by the name of Wilbur O. Atwater. He used a machine called a bomb calorimeter to combust a food in order to measure the heat—or energy—that's released. Needless to say, this is not how we digest food. More recent research shows that in certain foods, like nuts, not all of the calories listed are absorbed. For example, the calories of almonds were overestimated by 32 percent.[27] At the same time, the calories of other foods may be underestimated, especially those of vegetables and other carbohydrate foods, where different types of fiber and carbohydrates are absorbed differently.[28] Cooking, in and of itself, as well as the methods of cooking can also change the energy availability of a food. There are also user errors; it's easy to overestimate—or more likely underestimate—how much you are eating.

1. TASTE HUNGER
This is when you're not physically hungry but find eating a food pleasurable, such as ordering something from the dessert menu after a satisfying main course.

2. EMOTIONAL HUNGER
Desiring food to soothe or comfort an uncomfortable emotion, such as baking your mom's famous chocolate cake when you're feeling lonely and missing your family.

3. PRACTICAL HUNGER
Eating when you're not hungry because you're not sure when you are going to get access to food again, such as having a snack before going into a long meeting.

The hunger and fullness scale is a tool that's commonly used in intuitive eating to get back in touch with your body's cues and what it feels like to "eat in the middle." Below is how I describe the different levels of hunger and fullness.

THE HUNGER AND FULLNESS SCALE

10. BINGE FULL — Being so full you feel extremely physically ill or nauseous

9. THANKSGIVING DAY FULL — Being uncomfortably full to the point of indigestion or not wanting to do anything aka "food coma"

8. SLIGHTLY UNCOMFORTABLE — Having the feeling you usually do after eating a rich meal when you may want to unbutton your jeans or change into sweatpants

7. SATISFIED, BUT NOT STUFFED — Feeling full and satiated, but not physically uncomfortable

6. FILLING UP, BUT NOT FULL — Being hungry no longer but not yet satisfied

5. NEUTRAL — Feeling how you might feel a couple hours after a satisfying meal with your stomach feeling neither full nor empty and you living your life, not thinking about food

4. SNACK HUNGRY — Feeling a mild emptiness in your stomach or experiencing a slight dip in energy and finding the idea of a snack appealing

3. MEAL HUNGRY — Being hungry with your stomach feeling empty and perhaps growling, ready for a meal but not uncomfortable

2. UNCOMFORTABLY HUNGRY — Having stomach pangs and experiencing fatigue, aka being "hangry"

1. EXTREMELY HUNGRY — Being so hungry that you're feeling dizzy and nauseous and having headaches

These descriptions serve as a helpful starting point, but individuals may experience hunger or fullness cues differently. Check in with the hunger and fullness scale at random times throughout the day outside of mealtime as well as in the beginning, middle, and toward the end of the meal and take note of the difference in how you feel.

Besides a history of dieting, there are other things that can dysregulate hunger and fullness cues. Skipping meals or going too long without eating can also affect hunger and fullness cues. Gastrointestinal issues can make stomach cues difficult to feel or interpret. Acute stress can suppress appetite, as the fight-or-flight response releases hormones, like noradrenaline, which reduces appetite, and other catecholamines, which reduce blood flow to the gut.[29] Intense exercise may also dysregulate cues. Research has shown that the levels of peptide YY, an appetite suppressing hormone, increase for up to two to three hours after aerobic exercise, which is a time period in which nourishment is recommended to replenish liver glycogen stores and help rebuild muscles.[30]

In these cases, while appetite may be suppressed and you may not feel hungry, your body is still using energy, and it still needs food. If you don't eat, your appetite is often much stronger when it comes back, making up for what was missed—often more. This is why it's helpful to pair *body knowledge* (i.e., hunger and fullness cues) with brain knowledge of what may be impacting your cues.

Some examples of how body knowledge and brain knowledge work together:

"I'm not feeling very hungry after that hard run, but I know I need to replenish my energy. I'll have this protein bar that isn't overly filling but has good nutrition."

"I have zero appetite after such a stressful morning, but it's past my usual lunchtime, and I haven't eaten since breakfast. I know if I don't eat, my brain won't be fueled, and it will just add to my stress. So, I'll take a quick break and grab something that's light on my stomach and comforting, like soup."

"Even though I've only eaten half of my usual meal, I feel uncomfortably full. I've also felt bloated and constipated all day, so that's probably impacting how I feel. I'll stop now because I don't feel great. But I should be prepared with a snack for a little later since I'll probably feel hungry again soon."

In these examples, your hunger and fullness cues are *clues*, not rules.

The idea of trusting your body may feel scary and confusing after years of looking to diets for guidance on how much to eat. Think of getting back in touch with hunger and fullness cues as reestablishing a friendship with your body; trust that your body is your best friend and that it always has your best interests at heart. Can you return the friendship and be there for your body by feeding it adequately throughout the day?

Unconditional Permission to Eat All Foods

INTUITIVE EATING
PRINCIPLES:

MAKE PEACE
WITH FOOD

CHALLENGE THE
FOOD POLICE

I refer to these principles of intuitive eating as the permission principles, as they are all about giving yourself *unconditional* permission to eat all the foods you enjoy, which is critical.

Many of the foods deemed "unhealthy" by diet culture are perfectly nutritious, and by not eating them, you're missing out on the nutrition—not to mention the pleasure—that they provide. Restricting food also has a "forbidden fruit" effect where the off-limits food becomes even more desirable. Research shows that trying not to think about a food just leads to thinking about that food more and may even influence food behaviors, increasing binge eating and cravings.[31] Even *thinking* about going on a diet or restricting can lead to overeating. One study put people who liked chocolate on a three-week chocolate restriction and found that it increased their intake of chocolate both before and after the restriction period.[32]

It can feel incredibly scary to give yourself permission to eat all foods. You may feel that you don't deserve a certain food until you lose weight; you may feel fearful of what other people will think about you or that you won't be able to stop eating some off-limits food. If so, know that your fear is very real and very scary, as it's rooted in prior experiences with food that have felt out of control, and I believe it's important to validate it.

The following are some examples of how to respond to that fear:

Yes, I've binged on ice cream in the past. It felt intensely scary, out of control, and shameful, AND I know that restricting ice cream makes those scary experiences more likely to happen again. So, I'll give myself permission to savor this ice cream tonight.

Yes, I snacked on chocolate cookies constantly the last time they were in the house, AND I was also telling myself I would go back on my diet when they were gone. Buying a box of cookies gives me a chance to learn how to eat them in a comfortable way, and to see what it's like to have them around when they're not being restricted.

Yes, I feel like I need to lose weight to deserve the foods I love, AND I know that even though I don't love my body, I still want to treat it kindly. And that means eating my favorite foods.

When you start giving yourself permission to eat all foods, it is very normal to experience a honeymoon period—"Donutland," as author and activist Jes Baker terms it—when you may be eating much more of the previously forbidden foods, reveling in the fact that they are no longer off-limits. This period can feel really scary. Many people enter into it only to turn right back to dieting. They're convinced that intuitive eating isn't "working" for them because their eating is

What if I Think I'm Addicted to Food?

Fear of being addicted to food is a common fear, as the phrase "food addiction" gets thrown around quite a bit. However, the science behind the whole concept of food addiction has some major flaws.

1. Most of the studies on food addiction have been done on rodents. Suffice it to say, we are not rats. Rodents are used in studies because they are inexpensive and easy to house, not because they are perfect stand-ins for human beings. Even if they were, rodents don't have a relationship with food the way that humans do. Also, rats are highly food driven. We need to put these animal studies in context.

2. The rats in these studies only showed "addictive behaviors" when given intermittent access to sugar or when energy-restricted. When given free access to food, they did not display these behaviors.[35] Actually, these studies are a better example of how restriction fuels bingeing than of food addiction.

3. Even though high-sugar and high-fat foods are typically implicated in food addiction, not one addictive compound has ever been identified. Sugar breaks down into glucose and fat breaks down into fatty acid. Once that occurs, the body can't tell whether it came from a doughnut or an apple and peanut butter. If fat and sugar were truly addictive, they would be equally addictive in all forms regardless of whether it was from a "healthy" or "unhealthy" food.

4. The Yale Food Addiction Questionnaire, a tool used to categorize food addiction in research, has some major problems, one of which is that the questionnaire relies on self-reported responses as opposed to clinical evaluation. This means it works better in identifying people who feel guilty for breaking food rules—typically chronic dieters—than it does in establishing food addiction as fact.

5. One of the explanations of food addiction is that eating an "addictive food" lights up dopamine (pleasure) receptors in the brain in the same way that drugs do. This is true. However, this is also the case with many other pleasurable activities, like physical touch, listening to music, socializing, and being outdoors. While it's true that food addiction studies show a dopamine response that had a similar strength as drugs, that response occurred only in the rodents that were deprived.[36] This makes sense because we know that restriction makes a food more pleasurable. Also, dopamine isn't the only piece of the brain's addiction pathway, and just because food can share one part of the pathway does not make it addictive.

6. If food addiction were real, abstinence would be the solution. However, for people with binge eating disorder, learning how to eat the foods they binge eat (and often believe they are addicted to) is an essential part of treatment, as building skills with these foods significantly decreases binge eating.[37] I can't imagine that being a part of any reputable substance abuse program.

I think one of the reasons we are attached to the food-addiction narrative is that willpower is normally blamed for overeating or bingeing. The concept of food addiction takes away some of that blame (i.e., it's not *you* that's at fault; it's the food). In truth, it's neither willpower nor addiction that's to blame; it's *restriction* that triggers these unwanted eating behaviors.

"out of control," not realizing the dieting is what caused the out-of-control eating in the first place. However, the honeymoon period is essential to healing your relationship with food, and there is no need to rush it. Just know that when you come out the other end, you will have built up trust that the forbidden foods will always be available. Eventually, these foods will be normalized to the point where they no longer seem so intensely appealing.

The process by which a food loses some of its appeal after you repeatedly expose yourself to it is called *habituation*.[33] This can happen over a period of time, like when you can't stand the sight of turkey after three days of eating Thanksgiving leftovers; habituation also happens as you're eating, like how a rich chocolate cake tastes like heaven at the first bite only to be cloying by the time you take the fifth bite.

However, studies show that habituation may be delayed by both distraction and stress.[34] So, as you are reintroducing a forbidden food, it may be helpful to try it on a day that it's not too stressful and aim to slow down and tune in to how your food tastes. Make sure you're not overly hungry so you won't eat it in a way that feels out of control. Start with a less scary food. Plan the forbidden food as part of a typical meal or snack; for example, having french fries as a side dish for your usual roasted salmon and broccoli meal or having candy for dessert at lunch. Introducing foods in the form of individually portioned packages, like small bags of chips or ice cream cups, can be helpful for some, although it can create feelings of restriction for others. I often encourage clients to stock up on as much of a scary food as they can so they feel secure that this food will always be available, which prevents the deprivation mindset from being triggered.

Many people, especially those with a diagnosis of binge eating disorder, may need support from a dietitian trained in intuitive eating in this process. If reading this feels overwhelming, reach out for help. You don't have to do this on your own.

However—and this may be obvious—if the reason a food is forbidden is that you are allergic to it or truly cannot eat it for a similar health reason, like celiac disease, reintroducing that food is not a smart idea. That said, you may still be experiencing a sense of deprivation. This can be challenging. In this case, I've found that it's helpful to reframe it as an act of self-care, reminding yourself that technically you *could* eat the food, but you don't really want to do that knowing how it would make you feel. This makes it a choice instead of a mandate, and this can be incredibly empowering.

In addition to giving yourself the *physical* permission to eat the foods you enjoy, you also want to give yourself *emotional* permission. This is where you need to challenge the food police, the negative and unhelpful thoughts that try to control your actions around food by imbuing morality to your food choices. The food police create an emotional restriction around food and a sense of deprivation and shame that fuels unwanted eating behaviors and backlash eating.

Cognitive behavioral therapy (CBT) can be helpful here. CBT is a common psychotherapeutic intervention that provides us with the skills to identify and challenge cognitive distortions (i.e., unhelpful, inaccurate, and exaggerated beliefs that influence our feelings and behaviors). The principles of CBT can help us when it comes to food as well. Inaccurate beliefs about food create anxiety, often resulting in avoidance or emotional restriction of certain foods—the consequences of which reinforce the initial fear, creating a vicious cycle that looks like this:

THOUGHT ⟶ **FEELING** ⟶ **BEHAVIOR** ⟶ **RESULT** ⟶ **BELIEF**

THOUGHT	FEELING	BEHAVIOR	RESULT	BELIEF
Sugar is addictive and bad for me.	*I'm anxious when anything with sugar in it is in the house.*	*I keep sweets out of the house.*	*I overeat sweets at social events and see that as evidence of my sugar addiction.*	*I always overeat sweets when I am at social events, so I must be addicted and should keep away from them.*

To teach my clients how to challenge the food police, one homework assignment I give them is to keep a food thought journal for a week. I instruct them to jot down what they're telling themselves whenever they feel anxious or stressed around food. Then we use the thought journal to practice reframing those thoughts in session. Here are some examples of how to challenge the food police by reframing your thoughts.

CHALLENGE WITH FACTS
Counter with evidence-based information about food and how your body utilizes it.
(Chapter 4 offers more evidence-based information about food and nutrition.)

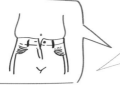

THOUGHT: "I shouldn't eat any carbs at breakfast; it will hurt my blood sugar."

REFRAMED THOUGHT: *"Carbs are my body's main source of fuel and the only source of energy my brain can use. Including a carb at breakfast will help keep my blood sugar steady until lunch."*

CONSIDER PERSONAL EXPERIENCES
Your prior experiences with food and dieting can be powerful evidence in challenging the food police.

THOUGHT: "My pants are fitting tight; I really need to do a cleanse."

REFRAMED THOUGHT: *"I've done cleanses in the past. Even though I lost weight in the short run, I've always ended up back in the same place. Perhaps I just need to put on a different pair of pants that would fit more comfortably."*

CONSIDER HOW YOU WOULD TALK TO A CHILD OR FRIEND
We often hold ourselves to unreasonable standards to which we would never hold someone else. Would you recommend that a friend or child eat in the same way you're expecting of yourself?

THOUGHT: "I'm not going to eat any sweets at that holiday party."

REFRAMED THOUGHT: *"Would I tell a child or a friend to pass on the dessert bar at that holiday party? No. I would tell them to look at what's available and pick out what looks appealing."*

CONSIDER IF IT'S TRUE FOR OTHER PEOPLE

You are not an alien. Your body works in the same way as every other human being on this planet. Barring food allergies and intolerances, food will affect your body pretty much the same way it affects everyone else's.

THOUGHT: *"I can't eat that burger. I'll gain so much weight."*

REFRAMED THOUGHT: *"I've been around hundreds of people who have eaten burgers, and they looked exactly the same afterward. Why would my body react any differently?"*

CONSIDER IF THIS THOUGHT IS HELPING YOU

Sometimes we make mistakes with eating. It happens. Is beating yourself up about it serving any useful purpose?

THOUGHT: *"I can't believe I ate so much pizza. I felt sick! Why am I such a pig?"*

REFRAMED THOUGHT: *"Okay, so you ate a lot of pizza. Is beating myself up about it actually helping? Time to move on!"*

TURN IT INTO A LEARNING OPPORTUNITY

One way to feel better about mistakes in eating is to turn them into opportunities to learn.

THOUGHT: *"Ugh, I can't believe I ate an entire bag of chips after work."*

REFRAMED THOUGHT: *"Well, of course, I ate an entire bag of chips after work! I only had a salad for lunch and got so busy I forgot to eat my afternoon snack. I was ravenous! What a good reminder to pack a more satisfying lunch and set a reminder for my snack because those chips ruined my appetite for dinner."*

REMEMBER THE POSITIVES

It's so easy to fall into the trap of bashing ourselves over the one mistake and overlook all the other positives. Make a highlight reel of your wins and replay that the next time you're feeling down.

THOUGHT: *"I can't believe I ate all that candy at work. I knew I shouldn't have let myself have sugar."*

REFRAMED THOUGHT: *"Yes, I mindlessly ate candy yesterday, but there are so many instances over the past few weeks where I've been able to savor sweets and eat them in a way that I feel good about."*

GET BACK TO REALITY

If you have a tendency to catastrophize or jump to conclusions, take a moment to bring yourself back to reality.

THOUGHT: *"If I buy that box of cookies I'm just going to binge on the whole thing and set myself off, and then I'll never stop eating."*

REFRAMED THOUGHT: *"This is an opportunity to build trust with myself by giving myself the cookies I've been craving. But is it really true that I'm going to binge on them? Even if I do, that one eating instance won't make or break my health."*

In challenging the food police, you'll likely notice that many of your food fears are directly tied to a fear of weight gain. This fatphobia, or fear of fatness, is often at the core of your food fears and restrictions. It is important to challenge the exaggerated fears over how food will affect your body size; it's also important to challenge the beliefs that make you feel fearful about having a larger body in the first place and to remind yourself that you would be just as valuable a human being at any size.

Treating Your Body Kindly

This theme of intuitive eating is all about being a good steward of your body by treating it kindly. The question with which I opened the book, of how you would take care of your body if you weren't trying to lose weight, has much to do with these principles.

The phrase "treat your body like a temple," a common trope in the wellness world, has always rubbed me the wrong way, but I couldn't quite put my finger on why. That is until I visited many beautiful historic temples in Japan and was struck by the attention to detail put into taking care of the temples and keeping them "pure." To keep the floors clean, you have to take off your shoes and not let your socked feet touch the dirty ground before stepping into the temple. You need to purify your hands with water before entering. I watched groundskeepers carefully raking the gravel walkway to remove every last fallen leaf. These are beautiful cultural practices for taking care of temples, but they represent an excessive level of care for something like our body, which is designed to take some wear and tear.

I encourage you to think of your body like your home instead. You get to decide how you want to take care of the body that you're going to live in for quite some time. Some regular maintenance is probably a smart thing to do, you can leave dirty dishes in the sink overnight or neglect dusting for a while, and it's not going to spell disaster. Rather than purity being the goal, as it is with a temple, focus on comfort, livability, and longevity.

Another way to think of intuitive eating is taking care of your body the way you would take care of someone else. When I think of someone I love and how I would like them to engage with health, these principles of intuitive eating all stand out to me.

Discovering the satisfaction factor is a principle of intuitive eating that often surprises many people. Pleasure is one of the most overlooked—and important—aspects of healthy

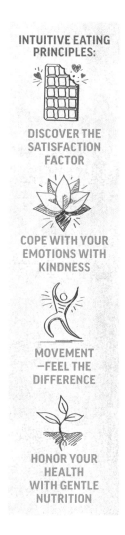

INTUITIVE EATING PRINCIPLES:

DISCOVER THE SATISFACTION FACTOR

COPE WITH YOUR EMOTIONS WITH KINDNESS

MOVEMENT —FEEL THE DIFFERENCE

HONOR YOUR HEALTH WITH GENTLE NUTRITION

eating. As human beings, we were designed to seek out pleasure from food, and the pleasure response that we get from eating has helped us identify important sources of nutrition.

That's why the phrase "eat to live" that gets thrown around sounds like nails on a chalkboard to me. When I worked as a hospital dietitian, there was a doctor whose nutrition advice to patients was, "If it tastes good, spit it out." I can't think of anything less empowering. The belief that healthy food can't taste good is a common one. When I ask new clients to describe what they think a healthy meal looks like, the responses are typically that it's bland and boring; plain oatmeal, baked chicken, brown rice and steamed broccoli, and sad salads all come to mind.

Fear of overeating tasty food is probably the biggest reason pleasure is so deprioritized in most people's attempts to eat more healthfully. However, we know that depriving yourself of what you like to eat rarely works out, as overeating and bingeing are fueled by deprivation and restriction. Surely, you've had the experience of craving something specific for dessert and trying to fulfill that craving with "healthier" options, like fruits, peanut butter, diet desserts, or dark chocolate until inevitably giving in to the thing you were craving in the first place. Can you imagine what it would be like to just eat the food that sounds enjoyable to you and move on?

This is not to say that every meal has to be pleasurable or satisfying. Sometimes we just have to eat what's available to us and know that more enjoyable food is coming in the future. However, when you have the option, it's helpful to go for what you *want* instead of what you think you *should* eat.

That said, years of choosing *should* over *want* can rob you of the ability to know what food you like. Intuitive eating can reunite you with your sense of pleasure, and that's a beautiful thing. If you're not sure what food sounds good, next time you eat, pull out the following list of food words and see if any stands out to you.

What Sounds Good?

TASTE:

☐ ACIDIC	☐ CRISPY	☐ FRUITY	☐ PICKLED	☐ SUGARY
☐ AIRY	☐ CRUMBLY	☐ GINGERY	☐ RICH	☐ SWEET
☐ BITTER	☐ CRUNCHY	☐ GOOEY	☐ ROASTED	☐ TANGY
☐ BITTERSWEET	☐ DOUGHY	☐ HERBACEOUS	☐ SALTY	☐ TART
☐ BLAND	☐ DRY	☐ HOT	☐ SAVORY	☐ TENDER
☐ BRINY	☐ FERMENTED	☐ JUICY	☐ SILKY	☐ TOASTY
☐ BUTTERY	☐ FIZZY	☐ MEATY	☐ SMOKY	☐ YEASTY
☐ CARAMELIZED	☐ FLAKY	☐ MILD	☐ SMOOTH	
☐ CHEWY	☐ FLUFFY	☐ MOIST	☐ SPICY	
☐ CREAMY	☐ FRESH	☐ NUTTY	☐ STICKY	

Taking care of your mental health is another way of treating your body kindly. Humans are emotional beings, and there is much to address within the intersection of food and emotions. A lot of stigma exists around emotional eating; it's either associated with a lack of control and emotional volatility or thought of in an almost comedic way as a young woman crying into a bowl of ice cream after a breakup. This shame keeps us trapped in the same behaviors. We need to understand that emotional eating is a normal human behavior. Besides, there are many ways of coping with emotions that are much more harmful than eating macaroni and cheese or a cookie to cheer yourself up.

Emotional eating can be a problem when it's overused because it's the only way a person knows how to cope. While food can soothe, comfort, or distract, it rarely solves the problem that's causing the emotion in the first place. So, instead of looking at emotional eating as wrong, think of it as one of the many ways to cope with uncomfortable emotions. Also, give yourself unconditional permission with food, because if you aren't restricting food, it is unlikely that food will be your preferred source of coping.

Some people who identify as emotional eaters meet the criteria for diagnosis for binge eating disorder (BED), which is the most common eating disorder. It is just as serious and deserving of treatment as any other eating disorder. BED is characterized by eating large quantities of food very quickly to the point of discomfort and feeling intense shame and guilt about it. With binge eating disorder, food is used to numb or punish rather than to comfort or soothe. If you think you may have binge eating disorder, remember that it is a mental health condition just like any other; it's not a lack of self-control or discipline. You would benefit from working with a therapist and a dietitian with eating disorder experience, preferably one who is aligned with Health at Every Size® and uses intuitive eating in their practice.

Movement is another way of taking care of the body. In the intuitive eating world, the word *movement* is used instead of *exercise* because it's broader and less associated with toning or calorie burning. While exercise brings to mind planned, structured physical activities with the goal of changing the body, movement includes unstructured activities and play.

Movement can be a beautiful thing with countless physical and mental health benefits. It can boost your mood, reduce your risk of chronic diseases, provide an outlet for you to bond with friends, strengthen your bones, help you get better sleep, and improve your body image. Unfortunately, exercise has become completely wrapped up in diet culture, even though research has shown that exercising more did not lead to greater amounts of weight loss even when calories were controlled.[38] In fact, it has been demonstrated that most people increase their caloric intake when they exercise, likely due to a combination of increased hunger and feeling like more food has been "earned."[39]

What's more important, however, is that when exercise is used as a dieting tool, it becomes joyless, robbing you of all the lovely health benefits that movement can provide. There's also a tendency to engage with it in an all-or-nothing way, like pushing yourself to do intense daily workouts only to burn out or injure yourself and spend the next few weeks on the couch recuperating.

Build a Self-Care Toolbox for Emotional Eating

The self-care toolbox is what I recommend to people who identify as emotional eaters. It's filled with a variety of tools you can use to cope with emotions. Certain tools may be more useful in certain situations, and different coping skills may be more or less useful depending on the emotion. Start by identifying what emotion is triggering the emotional hunger. Here are some common examples:

☐ ANGER   ☐ DEPRESSION   ☐ INADEQUACY   ☐ BEING OVERWHELMED

☐ ANXIETY   ☐ FRUSTRATION   ☐ IRRITABILITY   ☐ SADNESS

☐ BOREDOM   ☐ HOPELESSNESS   ☐ LONELINESS   ☐ STRESS

Next, come up with a list of non-food-related coping strategies. In creating your list, include tools that are helpful for processing, soothing, or distracting. Here are some examples:

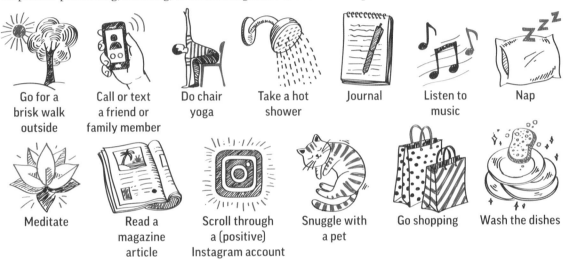

Go for a brisk walk outside

Call or text a friend or family member

Do chair yoga

Take a hot shower

Journal

Listen to music

Nap

Meditate

Read a magazine article

Scroll through a (positive) Instagram account

Snuggle with a pet

Go shopping

Wash the dishes

Now, add a few food-related options to your toolbox. Think about which foods help you feel better and in what circumstances. There's no judgment.

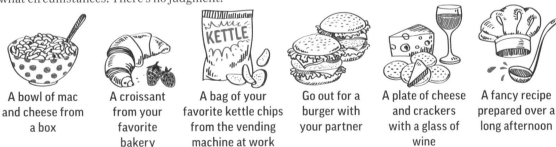

A bowl of mac and cheese from a box

A croissant from your favorite bakery

A bag of your favorite kettle chips from the vending machine at work

Go out for a burger with your partner

A plate of cheese and crackers with a glass of wine

A fancy recipe prepared over a long afternoon

When you're experiencing an uncomfortable feeling, look into your self-care toolbox and choose what feels good to you. Both food and non-food options are equally valid—there's no right or wrong. Keep in mind that if you end up choosing something that doesn't work for you, you can always return to the list and pick something else.

Vigorous exercise doesn't always promote health; in fact, instead of relieving stress, it actually puts stress on the body. Moderate exercise increases the levels of cortisol, the primary stress hormone, by 40 percent, and high-intensity exercise increases the levels by 83 percent.[40] Cortisol isn't always bad; it helps your body recover from exercise by repairing your tissues. Also, by putting your body through an acute stress like exercise and letting it recover, you can improve your health and increase your resilience to stress over time. However, without adequate rest, nutrition, and stress management, vigorous exercise can damage the body by increasing allostatic load, the cumulative wear and tear on the body, which I will explain in the next chapter.

As you can see, when it comes to movement, more isn't better. The Department of Health and Human Services' exercise recommendations for most healthy adults include 150 minutes of moderate aerobic activity or 75 minutes of vigorous aerobic activity or a combination of both on a weekly basis, along with strength training for major muscle groups twice a week. While this may be more than what you're doing or will be able to do—and that is fine!—it's less than what most people think they need.

Be intuitive with your movement and prioritize pleasure and fun. There are many other health behaviors that are just as important as—if not more than—movement, like getting adequate sleep, managing stress, going to the doctor for regular checkups, and getting your routine vaccinations. The only reason physical activity is put on a pedestal is because of its association with weight. Your body doesn't know whether you're riding your bike outside on a sunny day or riding a stationary bike at the gym; it doesn't know whether you're playing an active game with your kids or doing an aerobics class. You're still moving the same muscles and pumping the same blood. By putting more emphasis on pleasure—or, at the very least, on not punishing yourself—you're able to get the mental health benefits that come with it. Besides, you're much more likely to be consistent with movement when you actually enjoy it.

That said, there are times when it's helpful to "adult" yourself and engage in some movement like you take your medicine, like doing physical therapy to help heal from an injury, pushing yourself to go for a walk outside when you're feeling depressed, or doing a bit of strength training because you know it's good for your bones. But at least by decoupling it from weight loss and not punishing yourself with it, you can engage with movement in a healthier way.

Finally, the last principle that I've grouped under this theme of treating your body kindly is gentle nutrition. Gentle nutrition is the last principle of intuitive eating, one that I will cover in more depth in Chapters 4, 5, and 6. Gentle nutrition is not last because it is the least important; it's last because it's best to have done some work in healing your relationship with food and your body before you approach nutrition so that you won't turn gentle nutrition into a pseudo-diet.

The Journey of Intuitive Eating

It sounds like a cliché, but intuitive eating is a journey, not a destination. Its principles are here to guide your decisions on how to feed and take care of your body in a way that honors the nuances of your physical and mental health needs; they're here to help you tap into the resources that are available to you in the moment so you can make food decisions that you feel good about.

By recognizing intuitive eating as a journey, you'll also recognize that what you see as "failure" is just an opportunity for learning. Along the journey, you'll develop skills in the same way that you do when learning a musical instrument or a sport. It may be hard at first, but it gets easier with time. And yet no matter how far along you were in your practice, there was still more to learn. Likewise, coming from the diet mentality in which you're either on or off the diet wagon, you may find intuitive eating difficult at first, and it can feel like you're failing even when you're not. Diets, on the other hand, are just the opposite. They're easier at first. With rigid rules in place, you know when you're following the plan and "doing it right." But they get harder with time—much, much harder.

As you're healing your relationship with food and your body, you'll want to give yourself a hefty dose of self-compassion. We have all grown up in a culture that has an incredibly disordered relationship with food, and that's not something any of us has chosen. While you may feel frustrated by the many ways diet culture has shaped your relationship with food and regretful for having fallen in its trap, know that you were doing the best you could with what you knew at the time. Today, you have an opportunity to take a different path.

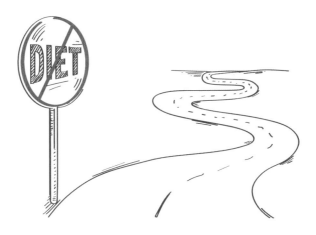

Chapter 3
REDEFINING HEALTH

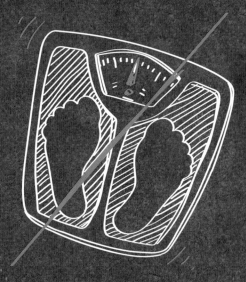

What comes to mind when someone tells you about their plans to "get healthy"?

My guess is that when most people say they are "getting healthy," they don't mean seeing a therapist, meditating, getting enough sleep, spending more time with family, driving the speed limit, getting vaccinated, practicing safe sex, purchasing better health insurance, getting a job that pays more money, or moving to an area with less pollution.

For most people, "get healthy" is code for losing weight. It means exercising more, eating less, and eating "healthier," according to whichever diet is currently in vogue. It may even mean following a rigid weight loss plan—often one that is explicitly unhealthy, eliminating entire food groups and/or requiring dangerously low levels of caloric intake. That's because health is viewed superficially as an outcome of food, fitness, and the number on the scale.

It's understandable. What do you see decorating almost every single doctor's office? A BMI chart. No matter your size, it's impossible to leave a visit without some kind of commentary about weight, whether it's a stern conversation about the need to lose weight or a reminder to "be careful" and not gain because your weight is okay now. Weight is hammered into us as the most important predictor of health. It's as if a "normal" BMI imbued some kind of immortality and a higher BMI was a death sentence.

For this reason, food and fitness are put on a pedestal as the primary means to improve health with the assumption that health is a personal choice, something you earn by getting every bite of food just "right" and sticking to rigid exercise routines. But health is not a choice, and weight is not an important determinant of it. Even if health was all about weight, the fact still would be that weight is more complex than diet and exercise, with over 100 factors influencing the number on the scale.[41] Yet the mainstream belief is still that weight equals health, which is why the misguided "eat less, move more" has become the prevailing motto for how to take care of your body.

I think it's important to look at nutrition in the context of a broader and more accurate definition of health so that we're able to engage with it in a more helpful way. This chapter, therefore, deconstructs the traditional view of health and redefines it away from food, fitness, and weight by examining its complexities and nuance and exploring its other determinants.

How the Traditional Definition of Health Fails Us

The definition of health is infinitely complex and nuanced. Ask twenty people for their definition of health, and you'll get twenty different answers. To further complicate matters, ask those same twenty people what being healthy looks like in their own lives, and you'll also get twenty different answers. How one defines personal health and decides which aspects of health to prioritize is not only highly personal but also inseparable from one's life experiences, culture, and the community in which one lives.

The way health is conceptualized has evolved over time. Traditionally, health was thought of as an absence of disease. This biomedical model focuses on pathology and biological factors of disease while overlooking the role which psychology, environment, and social factors play in determining health. In this view, health is binary: you're either sick or well. This model, which views the body as a machine that needs to be fixed (treatment) when it is broken (diseased), has a huge influence on healthcare as well as how health conditions are diagnosed and treated. It has also led to many of the complaints about Western healthcare for ignoring the role of well-being.

In 1948, the World Health Organization (WHO) developed a new definition of health, describing it as "a state of complete physical, mental, and social well-being and not merely the absence of disease or infirmity."[42] This more holistic definition was criticized as being too difficult to measure and too broad (if we go by this definition, almost everyone would be considered unhealthy). However, by recognizing the role of mental and social health, it represented a huge leap forward. Later, in the 1980s, the WHO started moving toward a wellness model, conceptualizing health not as a state, but as "the extent to which an individual or group is able to realize aspirations, to satisfy needs, and to change or cope with the environment."[43] Essentially, this definition of health views it as a resource that allows one to live an everyday life aligned with one's own values and goals and to cope with life changes that inevitably occur.

Despite these advances in how health is defined, the biomedical model prevails in the realm of healthcare—especially nutrition. You see this in the focus on lab values as well as in the prevention and treatment of disease. These things are certainly important, but they don't address the emotional, social, or community health needs. From the conversations I've had with friends, clients, colleagues, and those I've observed on social media, more and more people are experiencing this gap, and they are seeking resources that address their health needs in a more holistic manner.

These definitions aside, at the end of the day, personal definitions and views of health will always differ because everyone has different values, needs, and goals, which will never be captured with a binary view of health. Let's illustrate this with an example. Imagine an elderly retiree with type 2 diabetes and high blood pressure who suffered a heart attack five years ago. He spends his mornings being socially active in his retirement community, which is designed in such a way that makes it easy for him to get around despite his arthritic knee. In the afternoon, he generally rests or enjoys visits from his children and grandchildren, who make an effort to see him regularly, especially after his wife passed away a couple of years ago. Despite being "unhealthy" with multiple diagnoses, the man feels quite healthy and content in his life, and his chronic conditions do not interfere much with his quality of life.

Now imagine a young woman who is a recent college graduate. With a large amount of college loans to pay off, she is working weekends as a restaurant server on top of her 9-to-5, which is really an 8-to-6. It's a low-paying "starter" job, but she feels that if she works hard and does well, she'll have the opportunity to move up in the company. However, being so busy at work, she rarely gets to see her friends, and she feels lonely when she sees pictures of them together on social media. Also, because of her work schedule, she rarely has time to run, an activity she used to enjoy. She mostly eats takeout, which frequently upsets her stomach. And even though she has no medical diagnoses, she feels overwhelmed, exhausted, and quite unhealthy.

These examples highlight the subjective nature of health and the problem with defining health as the presence or absence of disease. It also shows how factors outside of one's control, like the environment, economy, and community in which one lives can have a significant impact on one's well-being. Yet, health messaging around us almost always focuses on individual behaviors, usually diet and physical activity. This leads us to believe that health is all up to us.

Granted, part of the focus on individual behaviors makes sense. After all, when it comes to health, there's not much we can do as individuals to improve air quality in our community or fix the economy. There are a lot of things that impact our health that we know are outside of our control, so we tend to focus our energy on the things we *can* control. Also, it's empowering to have knowledge that will help guide our decisions as to how to take care of our bodies. That said, this *inordinate* focus on individual behaviors makes it seem as if health were something entirely within our control; it also puts an immense pressure on us to always do the "right" things.

In reality, individual behavior accounts for only 36 percent of health.[44] And within that 36 percent, there's much more than food and fitness.

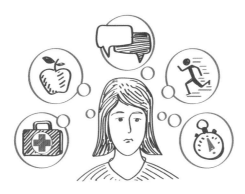

Determinants of Health

I rarely have a conversation about health with my clients without showing them this chart of the determinants of health. I find it essential to help put nutrition and physical activity into context for them so that they will be able to engage with these aspects of health in a more gentle and flexible way.

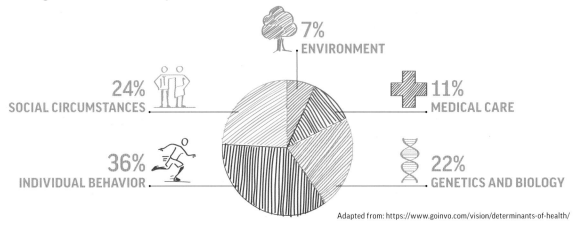

7%
ENVIRONMENT

24%
SOCIAL CIRCUMSTANCES

11%
MEDICAL CARE

36%
INDIVIDUAL BEHAVIOR

22%
GENETICS AND BIOLOGY

Adapted from: https://www.goinvo.com/vision/determinants-of-health/

Environment

This determinant includes all of the many health factors associated with the environment in which we live; it accounts for 7 percent of health. It includes factors in the natural environment, like air quality and exposure to environmental carcinogens, and the home environment, like the quality of tap water or exposure to tobacco use or firearms. It also includes community factors, like crime level, walkability, and educational and job opportunities.

The recognition of environment as one of the determinants of health reveals that many of the things generally believed to be outcomes of individual behaviors are actually outside of our control. I'll use my community as an example. My husband and I live in a middle- to upper-middle-class neighborhood, just a mile or two outside the downtown area. We also live right on the outer edge of a food desert. If you walk just a few blocks in one direction, you'll be in one of the lower-income neighborhoods in our city. For us, living in a food desert has never been a problem. I can hop in my car and drive just a mile down the road to an upscale health-food store, where I can conveniently pick up the ingredient I inevitably run out of while cooking dinner. Or I can drive a few miles further to my choice of five less expensive, yet well-stocked grocery stores. However, for those who live just a few blocks away, who don't have access to private or public transportation, there's nothing within a walking distance other than a couple of bodega-like stores and a very nice man who sells a few fruits and vegetables out of the back of his pickup truck once a week in the summer. For them, reliance on convenience foods is often necessary for meeting a basic human need for food. As you can see, many of the things we view as personal choices aren't necessarily a *choice*.

Medical Care

Accounting for 11 percent of health is medical care. This means having access to affordable healthcare providers with the appropriate equipment and skills to meet your needs. It also means having access to providers who are sensitive to cultural needs and able to provide stigma-free care, which is just as important. Access to medical care is a determinant of health that's often overlooked or underappreciated, especially by those with access to the medical care they need.

Furthermore, the lack of access to medical care can account for a lot of the health issues that are blamed on nutrition or weight. In fact, much of the association between certain chronic health conditions and higher weights can be attributed to how weight stigma affects access to medical care. Fat stigma is pervasive among healthcare providers, with countless studies showing high levels of bias among doctors, nurses, psychologists, and—it pains me to say this—dietitians against higher-weight individuals.[45] Providers often view the patients' weight as being largely a behavioral problem that stems from poor nutrition and physical activity.

As you can imagine, these biases affect the healthcare that higher-weight patients receive. Providers may also feel less inclined to provide advice on health behaviors if they believe their patients will not follow it. For example, a survey of over 600 primary care physicians found that more than half of them viewed "obese" patients as noncompliant.[46] Another experiment to assess fat bias in dietetics randomly assigned nutrition students to evaluate four patient profiles, which varied only in weight and gender.[47] Students who read the profiles of the patients with BMIs greater than 30 ranked them as less likely to comply with recommendations. Physicians also spend less time providing health education to higher-weight patients, despite the fact that they are more likely to blame their health problems on weight.[48]

Some of the stories I've heard from my clients are just heartbreaking. They've told me about the times when they saw their doctor for IBS or strep throat and, instead of having their symptoms addressed, were told to lose weight. Some clients, including ones who were in recovery from a life-threatening eating disorder, have been denied treatments, including knee replacement surgery, fertility treatments, and gender confirmation surgery, until they lose weight. Can you imagine how this might affect one's overall physical and mental health? A disturbing example of the poor treatment of higher-weight patients was the widely circulated 2018 obituary of Ellen Bennett.[49] After years of seeking care for the symptoms she was experiencing only to be told to lose weight, she was finally diagnosed with cancer. Unfortunately, at that point, the cancer was inoperable, and she was given just days to live. In addition, medical offices often lack the basic equipment to meet the needs of higher-weight patients, like comfortable chairs or blood pressure cuffs.[50] As you can imagine, when you know you're going to be treated poorly, you're less likely to seek out care.[51] In fact, some researchers believe fat stigma is a primary cause for the greater health risks seen with increasing BMI.[52]

Genetics and Biology

 Overall, genetics and biology account for approximately one-fifth of health. However, the degree to which this is experienced individually may vary, as some conditions are completely genetic. In most cases, however, genes alone do not cause diseases, but rather dictate risk. Because of genetics, some people may be at higher risk of certain diseases, and others may be protected regardless of their health behaviors. Pretty much everyone can think of someone who lived an incredibly healthy lifestyle but still got sick at a young age, or someone who lived a long and healthy life, despite engaging in behaviors that were seemingly unhealthy.

My personal favorite example is Richard Overton, who at the age of 112 was America's oldest living man in 2018.[53] Overton started each day with pancakes or a cinnamon bun along with several cups of coffee, each sweetened with three spoons of sugar. Throughout the day, he sipped Dr Pepper and smoked up to twelve cigars, followed by whiskey and Coca-Cola before bed. Overton's story makes me think of all the diet gurus selling a program that "worked" for them. I wish he had tried to make a buck with the Overton diet!

Social Circumstances

 This determinant of heath reflects the social environment in which you grow up and live. It includes culture, social connectedness, and factors that impact social status and experiences of discrimination, including race and ethnicity, citizenship status, income and education level, gender identity, and sexual orientation.

One aspect of this determinant of health that I like to emphasize is the role of social connectedness. In my ideal world, instead of commenting on weight, doctors would advise patients to call a friend, spend time with family, or volunteer. Human beings evolved to live in a strong community, and the role of friends, family, spouses, and neighbors continues to support health in our modern environment.

In the 2012 book *Blue Zones: 9 Lessons for Living Longer From the People Who've Lived the Longest,* National Geographic explorer Dan Buettner traveled to five areas around the world, which are known for their high concentration of centenarians, and studied why people in these areas lived longer and healthier lives.[54] Three of the themes he observed were engagement in spirituality or religion, healthy social circles, and strong family connections. For example, in Sardinia, family is considered to be the purpose of life, and in Okinawa, women have an average social support system of five other women, compared to two for American women. In these areas, spirituality, family, and friends are built into the culture.

Buettner's findings on the importance of family were corroborated with a 2020 study of Chinese centenarians, which found that 72 percent of them were visited by their family every day, and 95 percent ranked their relationship with their family as good or very good.[55] A study of Australian centenarians found that while their level of regular family contact was significantly lower than that of Chinese centenarians, their other social connections were stronger, with 59 percent reporting regular contact with friends, and 62 percent with neighbors.[56] Being around other people seems to be the thing that makes the difference no matter who they are.

On the other hand, research consistently links loneliness and lack of social connection to poor health. One study of over 9,000 older adults found that those with a lack of social connections have about twice the risk of death of those who have the strongest social connections.[57] Perhaps more importantly, strong family and social connections improve the quality of life and have been linked to greater life satisfaction, stronger resilience, self-compassion, optimism, self-efficacy, and self-esteem.[58] The fact that strong social connections improve both health *and* quality of life is one of the main reasons I like to emphasize the importance of this factor. After all, what's the point of a long, healthy life if it isn't also a happy one?

Individual Behaviors

 At 36 percent, individual behaviors are the determinant that has the greatest impact on overall health. Personally, I find this percentage comforting. It says that even though how we take care of our body matters, it doesn't account for everything. So there's no need to stress over always having to make the perfect decision. Some people might not be comforted by the idea that much about their health is out of their control, but, frankly, I feel that this has freed me from the kind of responsibility I wouldn't want to take on. If your health was indeed 100 percent in your control, would you be able to have any fun at all in life? Can you imagine the amount of headspace that would go into analyzing each and every decision?

When I talk about individual health behaviors, most people assume this means 36 percent of our health is determined by diet and exercise. However, individual health behaviors go far beyond food and movement. This determinant also includes sleep patterns, stress management, and risk-related behaviors, like motor-vehicle behavior, gun use, and drug or alcohol use. Though you're less likely to see these other factors emphasized, they are just as important as food and movement—possibly more.

Sleep, for example, plays a vital role in health. While you may think of sleep as being a time for rest, your body is actually doing quite a bit of work. When you sleep, your brain is busy organizing memories, while the rest of your body repairs tissue, grows muscle, and synthesizes hormones. Sleep deprivation has been linked to heart disease, kidney disease, high blood pressure, diabetes, depression, and more.[59] Just one night of inadequate sleep affects your hormones, including insulin, ghrelin (the hunger hormone), and leptin (the fullness hormone); this is one of the reasons hunger and fullness cues can feel wonky when you're sleep-deprived. As we have all personally experienced, poor sleep also affects mood, energy, decision making, attention, and motivation. Don't you find it hard to engage in other healthy behaviors when you're tired? After a sleepless night, all I want to do is eat takeout and lie on the couch.

Stress management is another factor. Of course, the number of stressors you have to deal with isn't always an individual choice. You could have strong coping skills, but that doesn't mean that life won't sometimes—or frequently—deal you a tough hand. This is not entirely a negative thing, as acute stressors can be adaptive and foster resiliency. However, when stress becomes chronic, it can overwhelm and impact practically every system in the body, including the immune, cardiovascular, gastrointestinal, musculoskeletal, and reproductive systems.

We live in an environment where stress is the norm; in many cases, our chronically busy culture even celebrates it. Yet, even with the knowledge of how stress is one of the determinants of health, we still often downplay its role while exaggerating the importance of food and fitness. You can see the hypocrisy in how we praise working parents for "doing it all" only to judge them for feeding the family with takeout pizza, or in how we admire wealthy entrepreneurs, who burn the midnight oil growing their business but look down upon working-class people for eating food from a box. As someone who likes to look at health

Allostatic Load and What It Means for Health

Allostatic load is the cumulative wear and tear on the body that comes from chronic stress. Stress isn't necessarily a bad thing. It can motivate you to do well in a presentation, figure out a solution to a problem, or get out of a dangerous environment. Physiologically, stress can help build resilience as you adapt to the stressor. However, when stress is chronic, and when your body does not have adequate support to recover, this leads to allostatic overload.

Stress activates the hypothalamic-pituitary-adrenal (HPA) axis, which is responsible for regulating the body's response to stress. The main effect of HPA activation is the release of glucocorticoids, including the well-known stress hormone cortisol. While cortisol plays many essential roles in the body, an excess of it from chronic HPA axis activation increases blood glucose, suppresses the immune system, decreases bone formation, dysregulates appetite, and affects sex hormones.

I like to use the bucket analogy to explain allostatic load. Think of your individual stress tolerance as a bucket. Some people have a big bucket that can tolerate large amounts of stress, while others have a smaller bucket. Now think of all the different stressors in life as ladles full of water that get poured into your bucket. When it starts to overflow, you experience symptoms of allostatic overload, which is when the stress on your body impacts physical health. Symptoms of allostatic overload might include migraines, insomnia, gastrointestinal problems, chronic pain, inflammation, or high blood pressure. To prevent allostatic overload, you can either lessen the amount of water going into the bucket, by reducing or removing the stressors from your life or by developing skills for dealing with them. Alternatively, you can pour a little water out by engaging in preventative maintenance and self-care, which I will talk more about in Chapter 6.

with a zoomed-out lens, I find all the focus on food and fitness quite frustrating, as it shows that what we're really afraid of is fatness and not poor health.

Food and nutrition can be a major source of stress, further adding to allostatic load. We eat—hopefully—at least three times a day, and if each one of these eating experiences is loaded with fear, anxiety, and uncertainty, you can imagine how that could impact health. In fact, the psychologist Paul Rozin, who has researched attitudes toward food in the US in comparison to those in other countries, has suggested that the worry over food and eating may have a worse effect on our health than food itself.[60]

And as for fitness, it absolutely does affect health. Physical activity's role in improving health and well-being is well established, and we know it's good for you regardless of whether or how it affects weight. A prospective study of over 80,000 people, spanning over thirty-five years, found that cardiorespiratory fitness was more protective than being at what's considered a "normal" BMI.[61] The takeaway from the study was that being "fat but fit" was healthier than being "unfat and unfit." Even better news: research shows any bit of movement counts. Even light movement, like strolling the neighborhood or cleaning the house, has been shown to reduce the risk of premature death.[62] You don't have to become an athlete to improve your health.

Nutrition matters also. Even though all the back-and-forth you see in nutrition headlines may make it seem like no one has any idea what to eat, we actually have good evidence of certain patterns of eating being associated with better health and longevity. The key word here is *patterns.* The big picture is what matters when it comes to nutrition, not the minor details over which the headlines usually obsess. These healthy patterns of eating are all about the very boring and unsexy nutrition advice you've heard a million times before: eat nutrient-rich foods (like fruits, vegetables, and whole grains), balance your plate (with fat, protein, and carbs), and eat a variety of foods.

However, within these patterns, there can be a wide variance in terms of macronutrient content and what individual foods are emphasized. When you look at dietary patterns around the world, you'll realize that people eat what's available to them. For example, a traditional Okinawan diet is 90 percent carbohydrate, while a traditional Mediterranean diet is over 40 percent fat. In Mexico, traditional dietary patterns include lots of corn, squash, and beans. Nordic countries eat lots of omega-3-rich fatty fish, berries, root vegetables, as well as grains, like barley, oats, and rye. In the countries of West Africa, diets are rich in greens, peanuts, spices, and starchy vegetables, such as yams and cassava. The wide variance of human diets around the world is evidence of our adaptability as a species. Human beings were literally designed to be flexible around food.

That said, nutrition is just one small piece of health. Certainly, good nutrition gives you a better *quality* of life, increases your energy levels, mood, and helps you feel better physically. However, there's no proof that there is one "right" way to eat. Even if science agreed on what that looks like, there would still be no guarantee that it would lead to good health or that it would offset the risks from other determinants of health. Stress, on the other hand—including stress over nutrition in the name of health—has been shown to detract from the quality of your life.

How Did Health Become All About Weight, Diet, and Exercise?

To understand how health became so wrapped up in weight, diet, and exercise, it's helpful to understand the history of dieting. It goes back thousands of years to ancient Greece, and the original word for diet, *diaita*.[63] The Greeks used this word in a similar way to how we often use the word *diet* to describe a healthy lifestyle, encompassing food, exercise, sleep, and other guidelines for self-care. Apart from the making yourself vomit and running around naked, the original diaita was mostly pretty reasonable stuff as far as diets go.

Since then, we humans have run through our fair share of fad diets. Who could forget Horace Fletcher, aka The Great Masticator, who recommended chewing food until it was liquid? Then there was John Harvey Kellogg, the doctor who founded a high-class health spa that promoted bland, vegetarian foods and yogurt enemas. He also invented cornflakes, believing that it would help prevent masturbation, which, as far as he was concerned, was one of societies great ills. Kellogg didn't come up with this idea all on his own; he was influenced by Reverend Sylvester Graham, inventor of the graham cracker, another food that was created to prevent masturbation.[64] And then there are celebrity diets, which have been around for as long as there have been celebrities: Greta Garbo's celery loaf and buttermilk with yeast, Marilyn Monroe's breakfast of raw eggs in warm milk, and Elvis Presley's "sleeping beauty diet," in which he slept all day to avoid eating. Wherever certain bodies have been idealized, diets have followed.

While weight and health have been linked for quite some time, the intense focus on weight as *the* predictor of health is more recent. In the early 1900s, conventional medical orthodoxy generally regarded higher-weight individuals as healthy and underweight people as sickly and potential tuberculosis sufferers. This started to change when the Metropolitan Life Insurance Company examined age, weight, and mortality rates from about five million policies in the US and Canada to determine the pricing of life insurance plans.[65] Noting an association between higher weights and mortality, the company used this information to create the "desirable weight" charts, which were published in 1959. This precursor to BMI allowed doctors and patients to look up the range that they "should" weigh based on age, sex, height, and body frame. Unlike the BMI charts of today, these charts accounted for body frame and age. However, despite being used for a diverse population, they were developed using data from a relatively homogenous population of mostly middle- to upper-class white males, the people who could afford life insurance policies at the time.

In 1972, Ancel Keys of Minnesota Starvation Study fame, advocated to replace the Metropolitan Life Insurance charts with Quetelet's Index (see box), which was then renamed as the body mass index (BMI). This change did away with adjustments for age and body frame. Now people were basically being told to stay at the same weight from the age of 20 onward, even though it was known at the time that as you aged, having a higher BMI was associated with a *lower* risk of death.[66]

Why BMI Is BS

BMI is ubiquitous in healthcare. It is used not only to provide recommendations regarding weight, diet, and exercise, but also, in many cases, to determine eligibility for certain treatments, like knee replacement surgery and organ transplant. Insurance companies can also charge you more for a higher BMI. BMI plays such a huge role in healthcare, but it's unfortunately not evidence-based.

History of BMI

The BMI scale was developed in the 19th century by Adolphe Quetelet, a Belgian mathematician and astronomer, who named it Quetelet's Index. Quetelet was interested in studying the concept of the "average man," believing the mathematical mean of a population to be its ideal.[67] In developing his index, Quetelet specified that it was not to be used on individuals, but rather for evaluating populations. He was not studying any relationship between weight and health. Furthermore, the scale and formula for BMI was developed using mainly younger, white, male, Scottish and French soldiers, who lived in the 19th century— not exactly reflective of the wide and diverse population that BMI is used on today. In fact, BMI has been shown to overestimate health risks for African Americans and underestimate health risks in many Asian communities.[68, 69]

Type of body mass

BMI doesn't distinguish between fat, muscle, skeletal tissue, or fluid weight. More muscle and denser bones are both associated with better health, but they also increase weight and BMI. This is why, based on BMI alone, many athletes, including most NFL quarterbacks, are considered "overweight" or "obese." Furthermore, BMI says nothing about the types of fat or fat distribution. Visceral fat, which is found around abdominal organs, seems to be more associated with cardiovascular disease.[70] On the other hand, subcutaneous fat, which is found just under the skin, may be protective and is associated with lower glucose and lipid levels.

Arbitrary cutoffs

Have you ever wondered why the BMI categories are in nice, neat five-point increments? It's not because of science. The BMI categories as we know them today, with a threshold for "overweight" at a BMI of 25, were originally adopted by the WHO. It was based on a report by the International Obesity Task Force, a lobbying organization funded by the pharmaceutical industry, specifically, the makers of two popular weight loss drugs. Their report found increased mortality risk for BMIs lower than 20 and higher than 25, however, this range was because they didn't correct for smoking. Having noticed that "ideal" weights were essentially in a five-point range, they continued the trend and set the other BMI categories in five-point ranges as well—all because we like nice round numbers. In the US, the WHO BMI standards were adopted in 1998, and the cutoff for "overweight" was lowered from 27 to 25. Millions of people went to bed one night categorized as "normal" weight and woke up the next day as "overweight" and at presumed risk for diabetes, hypertension, and cardiovascular disease. This change was made despite the fact that the research they cited didn't show a statistically significant relationship between BMI and mortality until BMI was above 40.[71]

Wonky formula

The formula for BMI is weight divided by the *square* of your height versus the cube of your height. That would work if we were two-dimensional beings. However, we are *three-dimensional* beings, and this fluke in the formula makes it less accurate for shorter or taller people. Quetelet set his formula this way because when he used height cubed, he wasn't able to get that bell-shaped curve he was looking for to identify the mean. So, basically, he changed the formula to make his data fit what he was looking for. Again, not exactly great science.

In the late 1990s and early 2000s, there was increased talk of an "obesity epidemic" following the discovery that Americans had gained weight in the century prior, with an increase in velocity beginning around the 1970s (interestingly, that coincided with the time more doctors started recommending dieting for weight loss which, as we know, leads to weight gain). On a population level, not only had Americans gained weight, but we had also gotten taller in that time, with men growing an average of an inch taller than what they were in the 1960s.[72] Gains in height along with gains in weight suggest an overall improvement in nutrition status. This is because hunger was recognized as a problem, and national programs were rolled out to address it. Also, the food and economic environment had changed quite a bit from the 1970s to 2000s. Energy-dense foods had become more available and less expensive, whereas fresh foods had become more expensive. At the same time, income inequality had grown, pushing low-income people, with less time and money for cooking fresh meals at home, toward these more energy-dense convenience foods. There was also a trend away from more physical jobs and toward the more sedentary office jobs.

Despite the hysteria, "obesity" rates actually began to level off in the early 2000s.[73] Yet, the "obesity epidemic" rhetoric has become louder than ever, reaching a fever pitch after 9/11 when concerns about weight were linked with patriotism and the war on terror. The Secretary of Health and Human Services Tommy G. Thompson urged all Americans to lose 10 pounds "as a patriotic gesture."[74] Surgeon General Richard Carmona referred to "obesity" as "the terror within," and in a series of speeches warned that the threat was "every bit as real to America as weapons of mass destruction."[75] Ironic, considering those weapons turned out not to exist, yet were used to justify a very real war.

These fears were fueled by a 2000 report by the Centers for Disease Control and Prevention, published in the *Journal of the American Medical Association*, which claimed that more than 400,000 Americans died of "overweight and obesity," a number that would soon surpass smoking as the leading cause of preventable death.[76] However, the initial report did not factor in confounding factors, and an updated version released in 2005 showed that "overweight and obesity" were actually associated with an excess of 26,000 deaths, with the "overweight" category actually showing a lower risk of death compared to the "normal" weight category.[77] Not only that, but the study found more US deaths in the "underweight" category than in "overweight" and "obese." Yet, we didn't see any thinness prevention programs rolled out. Unfortunately, this updated report didn't garner nearly the number of headlines as the original did, and consequently, we were stuck on the idea that higher weights were a major cause of death.

In 2013, the American Medical Association overwhelmingly voted to pass Resolution 420, which recognized "obesity" as a disease. This went against the recommendations of its own committee, who had spent the previous year investigating the matter.[78] The committee had argued that "obesity" is not a disease because of the flaws in using BMI for diagnosis, the fact that there are no specific symptoms associated with it, and the fact that many people who are categorized as "obese" are metabolically perfectly healthy. It's been speculated that money was behind the decision. Two new weight loss medications had entered the market in the previous year, and it was thought that classifying "obesity" as a disease could help with sales. Also, this change allows physicians to receive higher reimbursement rates simply for mentioning weight in appointments.

At the end of the day, the reason why health has become all about weight boils down to money. The more people whose bodies are labeled as problematic and who feel fearful and concerned about their health, the more weight loss drugs, bariatric surgeries, diet foods, gym memberships, diet programs, diet books, and supplements are sold. It's a $72 billion industry.[79]

This focus on weight has done more to damage our health than to help it. We've spent all this time, energy, and money trying to solve an issue which, as I'll discuss in the next section, doesn't matter much when it comes to health. Not only does the focus on individual weight management ignore the systemic issues that affect health, it has also created generations of people trapped in a cycle of yo-yo dieting and body discontent.

Weight Is Not Health

Let's get one thing out of the way: Yes, there is an association between higher weights and certain chronic diseases, like diabetes and heart disease. But correlation is *not* causation, a fact that seems to be forgotten in the discussion of weight and health. Weight has little to do with health. The assumptions that being at a high weight causes poor health and that weight loss improves health are built on bad science.

Consider the association between baldness and heart disease, as pointed out in the book *Health at Every Size* by Linda Bacon. While there is a link between baldness and heart disease, that doesn't mean baldness *causes* heart disease, and no doctor would recommend medications or procedures to grow back hair as a way of improving heart health. We are able to see that link and intrinsically understand that there is a confounding factor, something that increases a risk of both heart disease *and* of baldness. In this case, high levels of testosterone are likely the culprit.[80] Similarly, when it comes to the association between weight and health, there are many confounding factors that are rarely accounted for in the research:

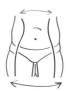

WEIGHT CYCLING
Also known as yo-yoing, weight cycling is the losing and regaining of weight from repeated weight loss attempts. Weight cycling has been linked to an increase in inflammation as well as an increase in cortisol levels, both major drivers of chronic diseases and factors that can independently increase weight.[81, 82] It is thought that repeated weight loss and weight gain as well as the ensuing changes to blood pressure, heart rate, and blood glucose leads to damage in blood vessels.[83] Some research even suggests that all of the excess deaths associated with BMIs greater than thirty could actually be caused by weight cycling.[84] Given our thinness-obsessed culture and fearmongering about weight and health, higher-weight individuals are more likely to diet and possibly more likely to engage in extreme methods of weight loss. This pressure puts them at greater risk for the health effects of weight cycling.

STIGMA

Earlier this chapter, we discussed the health effects of fat stigma and how it affects the quality of healthcare provided and leads to healthcare avoidance. Fat stigma may account for a significant portion of the excess deaths and higher rates of disease seen with higher BMIs.

POVERTY

Socioeconomic status is another factor that has been linked to poor health outcomes and may independently increase weight in some populations, especially for women.[85] One study found that moving from a neighborhood with a high rate of poverty to a neighborhood with a low rate of poverty decreases the likelihood of being at a higher BMI and the risk for type 2 diabetes, highlighting the role of environment in health.[86]

FOOD AND FITNESS

For some people, certain patterns of eating and a sedentary lifestyle may contribute to weight gain; for others, they don't. Whether or not these food and activity *behaviors* lead to weight gain, they are linked to poorer health outcomes. However, when these behaviors contribute to *both* weight gain and certain chronic conditions in some people, it's assumed that weight is the cause of the health conditions when, in fact, it's the behaviors.

Furthermore, the link between weight and health is vastly overstated. Except at statistical extremes (both high and low), weight is only very loosely linked to health and longevity. Not only that, but most research shows that people in the "overweight" BMI category have the lowest risk of death.[87]

So, what about all these studies you hear about weight loss improving health? Yes, there are many short-term studies linking weight loss to an improvement in *health measures*, like blood pressure, cholesterol, or blood glucose. However, it's impossible to know whether it's the weight loss, or the *behaviors* that led to short-term weight loss that are responsible for the changes. Since improvements in health measures usually happen pretty quickly in a weight loss intervention, before a participant has lost a significant amount of weight, my guess is that it's the behavior change that matters more than the pounds lost. I think the fact that behaviors matter more than weight loss when it comes to health is something that most health providers intrinsically know. If they really thought that health could be improved by weight loss in a vacuum, they'd recommend liposuction as a health intervention.

There are plenty of higher-weight individuals who are perfectly healthy, just as there are plenty of thin individuals who are diagnosed with chronic diseases. For me, one of the first chips in the mainstream weight-equals-health paradigm appeared when I worked as the dietitian for a cardiac unit, from observing how patients admitted for a heart attack were all different shapes and sizes. It was different from what I had been taught to expect in my weight-biased training. More than half of all individuals with a BMI between 25 and 30 are cardiometabolically healthy, as are 29 percent of individuals with a BMI greater than 30.[88] Furthermore, the focus on weight and health may miss the health risks and concerns in individuals whose BMI isn't in the "overweight" or "obese" categories, as more than 30 percent of individuals with a BMI between 18.5 and 25 are cardiometabolically unhealthy.

In other words, research has shown that the impact weight has on health is much less than what we've been told for decades. And the degree of that impact is not modifiable. No diet or other intervention guarantees sustained weight loss for more than a very small number of people. Not only that, but the focus on weight actively harms health. So, we have to look beyond the scale toward sustainable, health-promoting changes that enhance our well-being.

The Wellness Diet

So far in this book I have focused mainly on weight loss diets, including their negative effects on physical and mental health and the fact that, well, they don't really work as advertised. However, not everyone goes on a diet explicitly for weight loss. As diets—or at least talk of being on diets—start to go out of fashion, the *wellness diet* has popped up in their place.

Wellness is a nebulous idea that aligns with the more nuanced definition of health that goes beyond the presence or absence of disease. It encompasses spiritual, social, and emotional health and other aspects of health beyond physical health. While this focus on a more holistic view of health is all well and good, the wellness diet does not actually make us well.

The wellness diet is a term coined by dietitian and intuitive eating counselor Christy Harrison, which she defines as "the sneaky, modern guise of diet culture that's supposedly about 'wellness' but is actually about performing a rarefied, perfectionistic, discriminatory idea of what health is supposed to look like."[89] Think of pretty much every single wellness influencer, and you'll have a pretty good idea of what the wellness diet is. In its most obvious forms, the wellness diet shows up as detoxes, juice cleanses, and elimination diets. However, it can be much more subtle and insidious than that. Food as medicine, "clean eating" and the glorification of what's "natural," hydration as a trend, and an obsessive focus on yoga are among the more subtle markers of the wellness diet.

Compared to the "skinny at all costs" message of traditional diets, the wellness diet can feel positive and almost refreshing. But that's also what makes it so dangerous. The slick, filtered images and cheery messages of thin, young women with $50 water bottles and designer athleisure are a vision of health and wellness that is inaccessible to most people. It turns wellness into something that's performative rather than health-enhancing. It turns wellness into a trend you can buy into—something that's more about status and social signaling than about health.

In fact, some of the most fearmongering messages about food and nutrition come from wellness culture. In a world where being thin, young, and attractive is more important than professional credentials, nutrition pseudo-science—as you can imagine—runs rampant in the wellness diet. The hysteria over gluten, grains, innocuous food additives, or sugar supposedly has its focus on health, but the fear that it has created is just as harmful as the fear created by diet culture. Instead of telling you a food will cause your weight to go up overnight, the wellness diet convinces you that your body hasn't evolved to digest it or tells you that it will put toxins into your body or cause inflammation. It creates this idea that every single food you eat needs to be as nutrient-rich as possible; otherwise, you're doing it wrong.

Despite its claims to be about health and not about dieting, the wellness diet *is* a diet. Or at least, that's the intention behind it. Knowing that as we've gotten wise to more overt diets and their lack of long-term success, the diet industry had to rebrand its message to be a bit more subtle. That's why you see things like Weight Watchers' recent name change to WW, with the tagline "Wellness that Works," or food brands marketing their products as "high in protein" and "made with all clean ingredients," instead of "sugar-free," "fat-free," or "lite." Market research has shown the consumer shift toward wellness, and the diet industry has been more than happy to change its language to sell more products and plans. But that's just a bait and switch. Even though the language has changed, all of the most dangerous aspects of diet culture—the rigid food rules, the myth of us having control over our health or body size, and a vision of health that's off-limits for most—remain behind the facade of wellness.

As you can see, the wellness diet is not about promoting health; it's about scaring you and trying to convince you that you're not doing enough for your health. All of this is so that you'll buy more products. But, no, health and wellness can't be found in a pair of $100 leggings, a bottle of green juice, or a meditation app. While some of these wellness products may be enjoyable—and sometimes even useful—more often than not, they are a distraction from actual health and wellness.

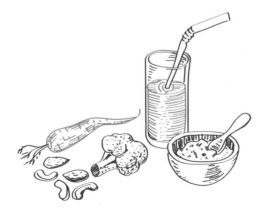

What Is Health?

If there's one takeaway from this chapter, it's that health is incredibly complex. Boiling it down to being all about food, fitness, and weight is missing the forest for the trees. Obsessing about these things makes us overlook other opportunities to take care of our bodies. Not only that, but it sends the message that all responsibility for health is on the individual, instead of looking at bigger systems that have a greater impact on societal health.

When I look at the research, it's clear to me that there is no single way of eating that guarantees good health, and anyone who tells you differently is lying and likely trying to sell you something. The idea of the "perfect" diet is a distraction from health. It pushes people toward engaging in drastic behaviors that are impossible to maintain, when, instead, they could be putting their energy into forming sustainable habits with food, movement, and lifestyle. Worse, many of these behaviors, rooted in an attempt to fight biology and manipulate the scale, actively harm us by causing stress and negatively impacting other areas of health.

We've learned about what health isn't, as well as the various myths and distractions that have long clouded our understanding of what health really is. But what, then, is health? Through the lens of intuitive eating, I have found a few things to be true about health.

Health is not a state of being; it's a resource—a physical, mental, social, and community resource that allows you to live a quality life that is in line with your values and goals. Health is not static either; it is a resource to which you may have more or less access at different points as your life and your body inevitably change. And considering the determinants of health, you can see that access to health is neither entirely within your control nor your sole responsibility. However, while much of our access to health is predetermined or outside of our control, we can optimize access to health both for ourselves and for others in our community through the behaviors we engage in and the choices we make.

That said, the pursuit of health is not a moral obligation. You are free to decide how you would like to pursue health in your own life—or even whether that's a pursuit you want to engage in at all. However, I think everyone wants to feel good in their day-to-day life. When we recognize that health-promoting behaviors are *not* rigid ways of eating, militant exercise, or an obsessive focus on weight loss, it brings the pursuit of health back down to earth and makes it more accessible for everyone. You deserve the opportunity to improve your health without trying to change your body size.

While gentle nutrition is not a guarantee of health, it is one of many tools that can help in accessing greater health. Gentle nutrition isn't something that should create stress in your life or make you feel deprived, but something that should help you feel better in the here and now. It also shouldn't inhibit or compromise other aspects or dimensions of health, for example by creating stress or a barrier to connecting with others over food. Rather, gentle nutrition enhances these aspects of health. Putting the pursuit of the perfect diet aside makes space for you to learn what helps you feel healthier—physically, mentally, and socially.

Chapter 4
GENTLE NUTRITION

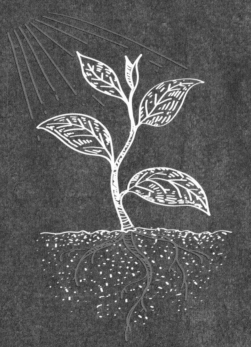

Gentle nutrition is, at the same time, the nutrition you always hear about and the nutrition you never hear about. It's the nutrition you always hear about because it encompasses a lot of the basic things you already know about food and nutrition; it's the nutrition you never hear about because it often gets glossed over in favor of flashy, fearmongering headlines. We have a bias for the new and exciting, and the media knows how to exploit that bias. So, when a new study comes out, no matter how small or poorly constructed it is, it makes headlines. The more fear these headlines invoke or the more they go against conventional thinking, the more clicks they get. This aligns with diet culture and its relentless search for the next new thing.

You can see that the way nutrition information—accurate or not—is shared is anything but gentle; it's rigid, prescriptive, and often framed in a way that preys upon your deepest fears and stokes your anxiety, instead of something that can be used in a positive, health-enhancing way. Think of the constant back-and-forth over whether a food is "healthy" or not, or the almost-magical powers ascribed to individual foods as if a single food has the ability to cause or cure disease. There's an obsessive focus on minor differences in nutrition facts, as if taking in thirty calories here or four grams of fat there really matters in the grand scheme of things. Mainstream nutrition is full of strict rules about what, when, and how much to eat—rules that require a massive amount of planning to stick to. It all makes nutrition seem exhausting.

Gentle nutrition is nothing like that. It can be hard to define because nutrition is so individualized, but essentially, gentle nutrition is about self-care, not self-control; it is about using nutrition in a positive way to take care of your body instead of punishing it. Gentle nutrition probably looks like how you would feed someone you love. You'd want to put some thought and care into nutrition, but you'd also want to feed them food that they enjoy and see them experience pleasure in eating. It is this kind of nurturing mindset that I want you to hold as we explore gentle nutrition.

Gentle nutrition looks different for everyone, depending on your needs, lifestyle, access to food, and preparation skills. What it looks like to you also can change according to the seasons of your life. Gentle nutrition may be a higher or lower priority at different times, and you're allowed to change how you approach it depending on your circumstances. Imagine how the incorporation of nutrition might look different for a sleep-deprived new parent than for a recent college graduate who's just learning how to cook, or for a runner training for their next marathon.

Gentle nutrition can accommodate your ever-changing needs because it is all about the big picture that's made up of little things you do over time to take care of your body. In the last chapter, I introduced the concept of dietary patterns versus diets. This is helpful to keep in mind as you go through this chapter, as gentle nutrition is about building health-promoting habits by making small tweaks and improvements to your personal dietary pattern.

To better illustrate the concept of a dietary pattern, I like to use a plane analogy. Imagine you are sitting in the window seat of a plane. On the tarmac, pretty much all you can see is the runway. As the takeoff begins, your field of view expands, and you can see parts of the city—buildings, car-filled parking lots, and roads. Once the plane reaches flying altitude, you can really see the patterns in what's around you—city blocks, neighborhoods, rivers and lakes, parks, farmland, and so on. The buildings, parking lots, and roads that you could see just after takeoff don't mean much in the grand scheme of your view.

Now, think about doing this with nutrition—zooming out from a few individual meals and snacks and looking at weeks, months, and years of eating. For all the worry about individual meals and snacks, as if they could make or break health, do they really matter in the context of a month? What about a year? What about a lifetime of eating?

Another difference with gentle nutrition is that it focuses on addition, not subtraction. Diets emphasize what not to eat—no gluten, no sugar, no grains, and so on. In practicing gentle nutrition, you focus on adding in nutrient-rich foods. For example, instead of telling you to cut out processed foods, gentle nutrition says to eat more fresh foods. Instead of telling you to eliminate white bread and pasta, it says to emphasize whole grains. This simple shift in mindset takes away the sense of deprivation and feels a lot more approachable.

With gentle nutrition, there's no either-or when it comes to food choices. There are no right or wrong choices; there is simply an array of options, some of which may be better suited to your needs than others, depending on the situation. When you look beyond the binary of black and white—of restriction and chaos in the realm of dieting—a world of flexible structure and gentle nutrition opens up.

Just as intuitive eating isn't all about doughnuts, pizza, and ice cream, gentle nutrition isn't all about fruits, vegetables, smoothies, and salads. As you make peace with previously off-limits foods, you're also making peace with "health" foods, thereby creating space for yourself to enjoy them both for pleasure and for the gentle nutrition they provide.

People often want to know what gentle nutrition looks like or whether they are practicing it. The thing is, because gentle nutrition doesn't look a certain way, it's impossible to know whether someone is practicing gentle nutrition just by looking at what they eat. It's as much about the mindset with which you approach nutrition as it is about your actual eating behaviors, and that isn't something you can see on the plate.

This chapter is all about helping you understand what gentle nutrition looks like for *you*. It will help you reframe nutrition away from diet mentality by unlearning all the diet advice and nutrition myths that have created stress around food and eating; it will also help you relearn evidence-based nutrition in order to feel confident in making food choices in a more flexible and approachable way.

Nutrition Hierarchy of Needs: A New Way to Conceptualize Nutrition

A couple years ago, on a trip I took with a group of dietitians, we had a long conversation over lunch about our frustrations with the challenges in communicating nutrition information to the public. In our conversation, a dietitian friend of mine pointed out how the media, and, therefore, the general public spend far too much time focusing on "high-level" nutrition while overlooking the basics. Articles on the ten healthiest protein bars, newest "superfood," and ten anti-inflammatory foods you must eat get churned out by the media outlets. Tens of thousands of people read them and start to believe that paying attention to these little details is important for health. If someone's interested in learning, that information is fine. In the grand scheme of things, though, it really doesn't matter if they eat the sixth healthiest protein bar or the first (or one that didn't make the list), or if they never have a chance to try the latest exotic "superfood." When people obsess over these minor details, they often overlook the aspects of nutrition that really *do* matter.

When my friend made this point, it was like a light bulb went off. I thought of all the times when my clients and my friends had asked me if they were eating the right breakfast cereal, or when they had asked me for my thoughts on what to add to their smoothie to make it healthier. Rarely had anyone asked me how to know if they were eating enough or whether they were getting a good variety of food.

That conversation inspired me to create what I call the *Nutrition Hierarchy of Needs.* It's based on Maslow's hierarchy of needs, a concept in psychology, proposed by Abraham Maslow, stating that people need to have their basic needs, like food, sleep, and shelter, met before they are able to meet higher-level needs, like a sense of belonging, esteem, and, finally, self-actualization. It's also based on dietitian Ellyn Satter's *Hierarchy of Food Needs*, which focuses on food access.[90] My nutrition hierarchy of needs isn't scientifically validated or published in any journals, but it's a helpful framework that I like to use with my clients to bring it back to the basics.

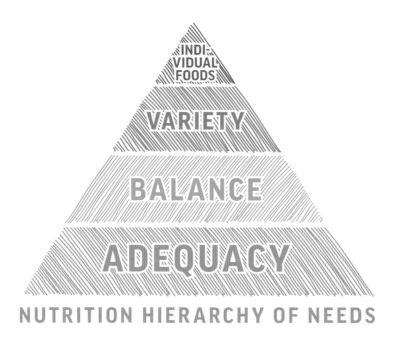

NUTRITION HIERARCHY OF NEEDS

Adequacy

By far the most important aspect of nutrition is whether or not you are eating enough. It doesn't matter how much kale and salmon or how many blueberries you eat; if you're not taking in enough energy, any theorized benefits that you're hoping to reap from their nutrients will be wiped away, as your body will use them toward your most basic bodily function of staying alive. Undernourishment actually stresses the body and contributes to allostatic overload and inflammation to the extent that no amounts of anti-inflammatory foods will be able to compensate for. Calories, macronutrients, vitamins, and minerals all play unique and vital roles in the body, and when your body isn't getting enough of those, it will suffer.

It's a common misconception that only those suffering from an eating disorder do not eat enough. The truth is that anyone could be eating inadequately with or without an eating disorder, and with or without them realizing it. In my professional experience, not eating enough is fairly common; it's at the root of many health and eating concerns. There's a lot of talk about how restaurants have normalized larger portions of food, and to a degree, that is true. However, at the same time, diet culture has also normalized minuscule portions of food. Consider all those frozen diet meals with fewer than 300 calories, or those tiny meal-replacement bars that people have been led to believe represent an appropriate amount of food for a meal. With diet culture influencing our perception of what a healthy meal looks like, many people end up not fueling their body adequately throughout the day, and they experience binge eating, fluctuations in blood glucose, anxiety, fatigue, and digestive issues as a result.

Another misconception is that those in a higher-weight body must be eating enough. The truth is that you could be higher weight and still be undereating. In fact, you likely have higher needs than someone in a smaller body does, even though society has probably taught you to eat less than them to "control" your weight. Eating less than what your body needs is harmful regardless of your weight. The size of your body might differ from those of others, but since your body functions in pretty much the same way as everyone else's, what's harmful to someone in a smaller body is harmful to you as well.

Keep in mind also that even though you may be eating adequately overall, a chaotic eating pattern—not enough during the day and larger quantities at night—can have a stressful effect on the body in the similar way as not eating enough does. Whether the inadequate eating during the day is intentional or unintentional (due to a busy and stressful work schedule, for example), it will be difficult for you to work on other areas of nutrition when your food choices are driven by primal hunger. So, I'd encourage you to focus on eating enough during the day as opposed to trying to tamp down eating at night.

At this point, you may be wondering how to know if you're eating enough. Unfortunately, there are no hard-and-fast rules. That said, there are some clues you can look for. Your energy level is one of them. It's very normal to feel tired from time to time or to hit a bit of a slump at certain times of the day. But in the absence of a chronic condition or other factors that impact your energy level, you should have enough energy to do the things you want to do most of the time if you are adequately nourished. Other possible signs include poor digestion, anxiety or depression, irritation, difficulty concentrating, anemia, hair loss, amenorrhea (loss of period), low sex drive, and many more.

With intuitive eating, hunger and fullness cues will also let you know if you're eating enough; you just need to listen to your body. However, if your hunger and fullness cues are dysregulated, practicing eating a reasonable amount of food throughout the day will help you reestablish them (see Chapter 6 for guidance).

Balance

 How many times have you heard someone announce their intention to eat a salad for dinner after having had pizza for lunch, in the name of "balance"? This is not balance. Balance is not trying to undo something "bad" by eating something "good." Even if there were such things as good and bad foods—and there aren't—bodies just don't work that way.

The balance that I'm referring to here is achieved by aiming to include in most of your meals all three macronutrients: fat, protein, and carbohydrate—plus, ideally, a source of produce. Each of these macronutrients plays a different role in the body and functions best when the other two are also present. The debate between low carb and high protein and high carb and low fat and high fat ignores the fact that human metabolism was built to utilize amino acids from protein, glucose from carbohydrate, and fatty acids from fats, and to turn all three into energy. Given adequate energy intake, technically, you can survive on a low-carb, high-protein, low-fat, or high-fat diet. Human beings were built to tolerate wide ranges of macronutrients, after all. But are you going to thrive?

Missing or restricting macronutrients creates a nutritional gap that's hard to fill. Because different foods have different nutrients, by cutting out or limiting certain food groups, you're also limiting your sources of nutrition. A low-fat diet, for example, makes it difficult for you to get enough fat-soluble vitamins A, D, E, and K, whereas a low-carbohydrate diet limits the amount of fiber, including gut-friendly probiotics, as well as vitamin C, folate, and magnesium.

Likewise, the lack of balance makes it challenging to work on the higher levels in the nutrition hierarchy. Studies show that when you're hungry—whether it's for food, money, or other rewards—the brain becomes more focused on immediate gratification over future benefits.[91] Despite the intention to eat healthier, when you're hungry, it's going to be really hard to make a mindful and intentional choice around food. Instead, you'll be focused on getting energy-dense food into your body as quickly as possible.

In talking about balance, I think it's important to note that this is a "most of the time" versus an "all of the time" kind of thing. Remember, individual meals and snacks don't make or break health. Sometimes you're in the mood for a bowl of pasta or even a salad of lettuce, veggies, and chicken; you just need to be prepared for hunger to return sooner than normal, as without all the macronutrients present, the energy from that meal may not last as long.

Variety

 Variety is the next step up on the Nutrition Hierarchy of Needs. This means eating a wide range of foods within each food group. Different foods contain different nutrients, so eating a wide variety ensures that you're consuming the nutrients your body needs. Also, focusing on variety can improve dietary quality by bringing in more nutrient-rich foods. Consider this a nutritional insurance policy.

Take vegetables, for example. A common piece of nutritional advice given to children is to "eat the rainbow," but this is good advice for adults too. The pigments in produce represent phytonutrients that have different health benefits—red lycopene is good for heart health, purple-blue anthocyanins support brain health, and orange carotenoids are great for healthy vision and immune support. By eating a wide range of colorful produce, you're getting the benefits of each subtype.

Grains and other carbohydrates are another example. Eating a variety of them helps ensure that you're getting enough fiber, even if you don't eat many whole grains. If you don't like whole-grain bread, brown rice, or whole-wheat pasta, there are many other fiber-rich carbohydrate options: white potatoes, sweet potatoes, oats, farro, quinoa, beans, lentils, winter squashes, corn and corn tortillas, polenta and grits, wild rice, barley, and, of course, baked goods made with whole grains. Instead of forcing yourself to choke down food you hate, focus on variety to improve your nutrient intake and to honor your pleasure.

Individual foods

Health benefits of individual foods represent the aspect of nutrition you hear the most about yet matters the least in the grand scheme of things. How many times have you seen articles, or been given advice, on what to eat to achieve clearer skin, blood sugar control, lower cholesterol levels, improved digestion, or a stronger immune system? Sometimes there's actual science to support the claims. Most often, though, a claim involves a kernel of truth that's been totally overblown. And other times, it's complete and total BS. Regardless, while individual foods can play a role in health, if you don't have a baseline of eating adequately, getting a balance of macronutrients, and eating a variety of foods, an individual food isn't going to make a difference for your health. No single food is a magic bullet.

I'll use fermented foods as an example of why adequacy, balance, and variety are needed first. Fermented foods, such as yogurt, kefir, and kimchi, contain beneficial probiotics that can aid digestion. However, not eating enough, or if going long times without eating, disturbs digestion. This is because eat stimulates receptors in the stomach, triggering peristalsis, the wavelike muscle contractions that move food along in the gut. So, if you're not eating adequately, peristalsis isn't triggered, and this leads to constipation, bloating, and other digestive upsets. Also, if you're undernourished, your body will conserve the energy that it would normally spend on digestion, slowing the gut down.[92] Without getting a balance of macronutrients, like when you're on a diet that cuts out entire food groups, it's also easy to eat either too much fiber or not enough of it, both of which can disturb digestion. Think low-carb diets that cut out fiber-rich whole grains and beans, or plant-based diets that include massive quantities of vegetables. Eating a limited variety of food or cutting out food groups can disturb bacterial diversity as well.[93] Given all this, you can see that even though it's true that fermented foods can improve digestion, without a baseline of adequate, balanced, and varied nutrition, these foods are unlikely to be helpful.

There are many other individual foods that have science-backed benefits for health. Oatmeal is high in cholesterol-lowering soluble fiber.[94] Folate-rich foods, like spinach, lentils, asparagus, and fortified foods, can help prevent neural tube defects.[95] Fatty fish does seem to be beneficial for cardiovascular disease prevention and may even play a role in reducing symptoms of depression.[96, 97] Research has also confirmed olive oil's role in preventing and managing type 2 diabetes.[98] It's great to know about the health benefits that different foods have to offer, but let's not miss the forest for the trees by obsessing over individual foods. Besides, if you're eating a variety of foods, you're probably already getting these benefits.

Why You Don't Need the Nutrition Facts

If you were hoping to find recommendations on what to look for on the nutrition facts, I am sorry to say that you're not going to find them in this book. That's because I never read the nutrition facts, and I tell my clients, except those with a few specific medical conditions, not to read it either.

It's easy to get caught up in arbitrary limits when we look at the nutrition facts. As human beings, we were designed to be able to tolerate variable amounts of calories and macronutrients from day to day. Different foods serve different purposes, so, of course, you will see that reflected in the nutrition facts. Salad dressing is supposed to contain fat, and pasta is supposed to contain carbohydrate. Something that has fewer calories isn't necessarily healthier; it simply provides less energy, which usually just means that it won't keep you full as long. If a food is high in protein, it either contains protein naturally, like chicken or tofu, or it's been supplemented with protein powders (which doesn't necessarily fill you up as much as just eating a source of naturally occurring protein with your meal). Besides, as we discussed in the last chapter, these numbers aren't completely accurate.

It all comes down to the fact that we eat food, not nutrients. The information you're looking for on the label can be found by tuning in to your body and your eating pattern. Instead of looking at calories, focus on hunger and fullness cues to get the right amount of food for your body. Instead of looking at macronutrients on the label, balance your plate with a carbohydrate food and a protein food, paired with produce and prepared with fat, to ensure you get adequate amounts of all three (even though meals will naturally vary in macronutrient content). Instead of worrying about sugar content, make peace with sweets so you can eat them in a way that you feel good about.

Nutrition facts can occasionally come in handy, however, provided that you're able to look at them without getting totally wrapped up in numbers. For example, I'll sometimes look at the calories in a frozen or prepared meal to help get an idea for whether that meal alone is enough, or if I should have something else with it. Also, when comparing multiple foods that look equally tasty, it's not wrong to look at the amounts of added sugar in different yogurt brands or the amounts of fiber in different snacks. For people with certain health conditions, this can be helpful. At the end of the day, however, these numbers should only be used as just one piece of information in making a decision about food.

Gentle Nutrition Guidelines

With gentle nutrition, there are no hard-and-fast rules. Nutrition is used alongside hunger and fullness cues, taste preferences, and food availability to help guide you in making decisions around food. Making food choices in intuitive eating involves bringing together body knowledge and brain knowledge. Body knowledge includes hunger and fullness cues, how food makes you feel, your cravings, and your food preferences, whereas brain knowledge includes nutrition information along with things like food availability and an understanding of how things, like stress or lack of sleep, affect your body cues. Nutrition is not more or less important than any of these factors, but depending on the circumstances, it may be higher or lower priority.

This section discusses the general nutrition guidelines, as well as some tips, that will help you round out your decision-making toolbox. Please remember that food choices should not be made in a nutrition vacuum. However, bringing nutrition into your decision-making process in a flexible manner can help you fuel your body in a way that feels good both physically and mentally.

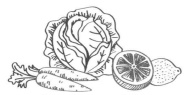

Eat fruits and vegetables

This is the most boring and least sexy nutrition advice of all time. But it's important.

Why do we nutrition folks keep nagging you about fruits and veggies? Because fruits and vegetables are loaded with vitamins, minerals, antioxidants, and fiber. They are rich in phytochemicals, chemical compounds found in plants—for example, allicin in garlic and onions, chlorophyllin in green leafy vegetables, resveratrol in grapes (and wine!), and capsaicin in chili peppers—which seem to provide our bodies with health benefits.

We have buckets of research linking the consumption of fruits and vegetables to health and longevity. A 2017 meta-analysis found a reduced risk of cardiovascular disease, stroke, and all-cause mortality associated with eating 800 grams of fruits and vegetables daily.[99] For cancer, benefits were seen earlier, at 600 grams daily. To put this in perspective, one medium apple is 182 grams, a cup of cooked kale is 130 grams, three cups of loosely packed romaine is 105 grams, and ten baby carrots weigh 100 grams. You can easily get this amount—if not more—just by including produce as part of a balanced plate for most of your meals and by including a fruit or vegetable as part of one of your snacks on a regular basis. But don't feel like you have to eat this amount of produce every single day. It's normal to eat lots of produce one day and little to none on other days. Remember, we're zooming out on patterns of eating, not micromanaging our intake every day. This study is simply a reminder that eating plenty of produce is beneficial.

Perhaps you feel a bit tapped out on fruits and veggies after years of chronic dieting. That's normal. Diets force you to fill up on huge amounts of fruits and veggies and often limit the amount of flavor-enhancing fat that you can use to prepare them. Of course, that will affect your enjoyment of fruits and vegetables. If you need to take a break from them for a while, that's fine. But when you're ready to add produce back in, be sure to focus on pleasure. Pair a fruit with some nut butter or cheese to make a satisfying snack. Use fruits as toppings for breakfast foods or desserts. Instead of steaming your vegetables, roast or sauté them with fat to enhance their flavor. Rather than treating vegetables like an afterthought, get creative with them, using different seasonings and condiments or adding things like cheese or sauces to them to boost the flavor. Try green beans braised in tomato sauce, roasted cauliflower tossed with tahini and herbs, or sautéed greens flavored with soy sauce and chiles.

Another barrier to eating fruits and vegetables is expense. Fresh fruits and vegetables can be quite pricey, especially those that are organically grown. It is perfectly fine to eat frozen and canned produce, which, in many cases, contain more nutrients than fresh due to the fact that they are typically frozen or canned shortly after harvest. While purchasing more organic produce may be helpful for the environment (which could be reason enough to buy organic, if you've got the funds), there does not seem to be a health benefit. Most people are familiar with the Environmental Working Group's "Dirty Dozen," a list of produce they have identified as having the highest levels of pesticide residues when conventionally grown. What the EWG doesn't tell you is that even though it's true that these fruits and vegetables come with more pesticide residues compared to others, the levels of the residues are actually so negligible that, as one study shows, conventionally grown fruits and vegetables are not any different from their organic counterparts when it comes to consumer risks.[100] Another analysis found that you could eat hundreds or thousands of servings of "Dirty Dozen" produce *every day* and still not experience health effects.[101] If you're still concerned, just give your produce a good rinse in water.

Eat whole grains and other fiber-rich carbohydrate sources

Whole grains are just as the name implies—whole, intact grains, or foods made from flour milled from whole, intact grains. This means you get the nutritional benefits of the bran (fiber) and the germ (vitamins, minerals, and fats), as well as the endosperm (carbohydrate, protein, and some vitamins and minerals).

A 2016 meta-analysis found that those who ate the largest amounts of whole grains had a lower risk of heart disease by 16 to 21 percent, a lower risk of cancer by 11 percent, and a lower risk of diabetes by 36 percent compared with those who ate the smallest amounts.[102] The analysis showed that even moderate increases in whole-grain intake reduced the risk of premature death. I love to use this study to empower my clients who have been subjected to the Paleo and keto fearmongering about grains.

Compared to unenriched refined grains, whole grains contain more B vitamins, magnesium, iron, and potassium. Whole grains also contain more fiber, which is helpful for digestion and better for blood sugar, especially for people with diabetes. For example, one study found that compared to white rice, brown rice had a 12 percent lower glycemic index in subjects without diabetes, and 36 percent lower for subjects with diabetes.[103] Because fiber slows gastric emptying (i.e., food leaving your stomach), you may notice that meals containing whole grains are more satisfying.

Why Nutrition Research Is Complicated

Have you ever wondered why the headlines on nutrition are constantly changing and conflicting? Part of it is because nutrition is a relatively new science, and researchers are constantly making new discoveries. But the main reason behind all the conflicts is that nutrition is a science that's notoriously hard to study.

For starters, we follow dietary patterns, not individual foods or nutrients. A lot of research makes claims about individual foods or nutrients, but researching them is, in fact, incredibly challenging. Adding a food usually means reducing or taking out another food and vice versa. To study individual nutrients in food, one would have to use a supplement, which may not interact in the body in the same way that a nutrient from food does. It's hard to know from studying food sources of specific nutrients whether a positive or detrimental effect is due to the nutrient, other components in the food, or the food itself.

To accurately study nutrition and its long-term effect on health, you would have to do a randomized controlled trial (RCT), which is the gold standard in other types of research, like medicine. In these trials, one group gets a treatment (the diet, food, or nutrient), and the other gets a placebo. To eliminate bias, the researchers are blind to who gets which. To ensure that the participants are doing what they're told and to monitor other factors, like physical activity, you would have to keep the participants locked in a lab and provide them with all their food. And because food doesn't have an immediate effect on health, you'd have to monitor them for the rest of their lives to see which group was diagnosed with more cancer, lived the longest, etc. Not exactly practical.

While nutrition researchers do conduct short-term RCTs, more often they rely on diet recalls and questionnaires, which ask questions like how often a certain food is eaten and how much of it was eaten. Of course, it's hard to remember what you ate for lunch yesterday let alone how many servings of tomatoes you ate last week or how often you ate dessert in the past year. Besides, given how food choices are moralized in the diet culture we live in, some people intentionally misreport their intake of certain foods. These questionnaires, therefore, aren't going to be the most accurate, which means the study results won't be the most accurate either.

Even if you could get an accurate assessment of intake, there would still be confounding variables affecting the results. Is higher sugar intake associated with poor health outcomes because sugar causes health problems or because people who eat more sugar tend to have lower incomes and be more at risk? Are people who eat more vegetables less likely to smoke and more likely to engage in other healthy habits? Researchers can try to correct for these variables, but it's not always perfect.

On top of all these issues with nutrition research, studies are usually reported on by journalists who have no training in data interpretation, science, or nutrition—and who, in an attempt to get coverage, tend to go off the press releases that often contain the most headline-grabbing findings.

This doesn't mean all nutrition research is for naught, but it does mean we should take individual studies with a grain of salt and focus on the big picture of what the body of research suggests.

Even though eating more whole grains is great, you don't have to eat only whole grains to be healthy. The fact that whole grains contain more nutrients doesn't mean refined grains are bad for you. Not every food we eat has to have a multivitamin's worth of nutrition. Refined grains still contain beneficial vitamins and minerals; actually, when enriched, they contain even more B vitamins and iron. In fact, you might want to choose refined grains over whole grains when you need a quick source of energy or when you want something to tide you over or take the edge off your hunger without making you overly full. (Think about how a little piece of bread helps tide you over until the main course when going out to eat.) Grains—refined or whole—are also a fantastic budget-friendly way to stretch vegetables and proteins into a more filling meal.

I encourage my clients to experiment with different whole grains to find out which ones they enjoy. To be healthy, you don't have to eat the nuttiest, grainiest, seediest whole-grain bread and have boiled quinoa every night. There are many products, like breads, pasta, and crackers, that are made with a blend of refined flour and whole-grain flour, and these are a helpful way to introduce whole grains. There are also several other fiber-rich carbohydrate sources, like beans, sweet and white potatoes, winter squashes, and corn, which are great foods to emphasize if you're not a big fan of whole grains.

Don't fear fats

If you were around in the 1980s and 1990s, surely you remember the low-fat diet craze. Fat-free cookies, fat-free salad dressings, and boneless, skinless chicken breasts were the health foods of the day—*blech*. Unfortunately, even though we've moved past that era (and maybe too far past it, since the latest diet craze has us swirling butter into coffee), there's still an aura of fear around fat—a fear that I'm fairly certain ties back to calories.

Yes, fats are higher in calories compared to carbohydrates and protein, but fats are also filling and make meals more satisfying. Receptors in the small intestine can sense when stomach contents are rich in fat; in response, they send signals that slow gastric emptying and release hormones that reduce appetite. The slowed digestion not only helps the body digest fats but also makes the meal more filling. Fats also enable you to absorb the fat-soluble vitamins A, D, E, and K.

The effect that different types of fat have on cholesterol levels is an evolving study which may seem difficult to keep up with. It used to be that most doctors and dietitians considered all fats unhealthy, then it became good fat (unsaturated fat) versus bad fat (saturated fat). Today, I could best sum up what nutrition researchers agree on with the shrug emoji. I think a lot of that comes down to the difficulty (and perhaps futility) of studying nutrients in isolation. Remember, we eat foods, not nutrients, so I don't know how beneficial it is to get into the weeds.

That said, here's my understanding of the current research on fats and their effect on cholesterol and heart disease risk. There are two main types of fat: saturated and unsaturated. Saturated fats are solid at room temperature, whereas unsaturated fats are liquid. One type of unsaturated fat, monounsaturated fat, is found in olive oil, nuts and nut oils, and avocados. Research pretty consistently shows that monounsaturated fat can lower cholesterol and that monounsaturated fat–rich dietary patterns, like the Mediterranean dietary pattern, are associated with a lower risk of heart disease.[104]

Another type of unsaturated fat is polyunsaturated fat, which includes omega-3s and omega-6s. Omega-3 fatty acids seem to be particularly beneficial for improving risk factors for heart disease, lowering blood pressure, and reducing inflammation.[105, 106] Omega-3 fatty acids are found in large quantities in oily fish, like salmon, tuna, mackerel, trout, herring, and sardines, and in a less biologically active form of omega-3 in flax, walnuts, and canola oil. One study that looked at 45,000 adults and estimated omega-3 intake through blood and fat tissue associated a high omega-3 intake with a 10 percent lower risk of heart disease.[107]

Omega-6 polyunsaturated fatty acids are found in margarine, seeds, and seed oils, like canola, safflower, and soybean oil. You may have seen the controversy surrounding claims that omega-6 fatty acids are inflammatory. While some recent research has suggested that consuming too many omega-6s in relation to omega-3s can contribute to inflammation, other large meta-analyses have shown that polyunsaturated fats actually reduce the risk of heart disease even more than monounsaturated fats do.[108, 109] This tells me that even if there is an effect on inflammation, it's small, and these mostly plant-based fats are generally beneficial. Remember that food is just one small part of total inflammation, so there's no reason to be fearful.

Saturated fats are typically found in animal foods, in the forms of dairy fat (butter, whole milk, etc.) and fatty cuts of meat, as well as some plant fats, like coconut oil and palm oil. In the past, people were advised to avoid these fats due to the belief that they are linked to increasing LDL cholesterol (often referred to as bad cholesterol) and risk for heart disease. However, more recent research has put that into question. A 2015 meta-analysis found no association between saturated fat intake and heart disease, stroke, diabetes, or death.[110] It may be that saturated fats increase cholesterol, but that doesn't translate to an increased risk of heart disease, which is much more complex than high cholesterol levels in the blood. While this research doesn't make butter out to be a "superfood," the way some nutrition communities have, it does say that there's no reason to be anxious about saturated fats. If you have a history of heart disease or are at high risk, you might want to be a bit more mindful of saturated fats. However, this doesn't mean you can never enjoy a steak or use butter in cooking.

My interpretation of all this research on fats is that fats are filling, they make food taste better, and they are an essential part of our diet. There is no reason to skimp on fats. I generally recommend that your everyday fats be plant-based fats, like olive oil, canola oil, and avocado oil, for both versatility and nutrition. However, animal-based fats, like butter, ghee, and bacon, are wonderful for adding flavor and creating a rich mouthfeel in cooking and baking, and you shouldn't be afraid of them. Enjoy fattier cuts of meat if you like, but also emphasize more seafood and plant-based meals. Don't hesitate to purchase full-fat cheeses, yogurt, and milk if you enjoy them.

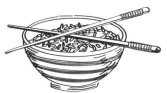

Eat more plants and fewer animals

Because addressing individual nutrients is so challenging, I find research on dietary patterns to be much more compelling when it comes to nutrition information. And in looking at research on healthy dietary patterns around the world, one general theme that has emerged is an emphasis on more plants and fewer animal foods—even if it's just a little bit fewer.

Dietary patterns of the cultures around the globe vary. We have heard quite a lot about the health benefits of a Mediterranean dietary pattern, but research also supports traditional African, Asian, and Latin American patterns. Each of these dietary patterns has variance within itself, and the foods emphasized therein are also different. Consider the difference between Vietnamese food and Chinese food or Moroccan food and Greek food. And, of course, there are regional differences within each country as well.

That said, if you zoom out on the traditional dietary patterns of the world, you'll find that they have a lot in common. One of the most notable commonalities is a focus on plant foods over animal foods. You can see this theme in staple meals consumed across all of these regions. Take beans and rice, for example—there's West African jollof rice with black-eyed peas, Brazilian black beans and rice, Indian dal served with rice, and Egyptian kushari, a dish of rice, lentils, and pasta topped with tomato sauce, chickpeas, and fried onions. Oldways, a nutrition nonprofit that promotes heritage-based diets, has worked with nutrition researchers, dietitians, and regional food experts to create African, Asian, and Latin American heritage diet pyramids, and each pyramid promotes an emphasis on more plant-centered meals.[111]

However, this doesn't mean you need to cut out all meat if you don't want to. While vegetarian and vegan diets can be perfectly healthy, research on flexitarian dietary patterns, in which meat and fish are consumed, though less often, shows health benefits, including improved blood pressure and a lower risk of type 2 diabetes.[112] So, if you enjoy eating meat, don't give it up. Animal foods, including eggs and dairy, are packed with filling protein and are the only food sources of vitamin B12. This is an area where it's helpful to focus on positive nutrition. Instead of thinking about eating less meat, let's think about eating more of the meatless meals that you enjoy.

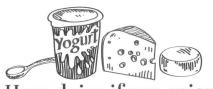

Have dairy if you enjoy it

After sugar, dairy is the food that my clients are most fearful about, as dairy has been so maligned in diet culture. If you were to believe all the bad press, then you'd think that dairy clogs your arteries, causes cancer, and destroys your gut, or that it is inflammatory and fattening, not to mention unnatural to consume unless you are a baby cow.

While it's true that many cultures do not consume dairy at all or only in very small amounts, and that we don't need dairy to survive, the fearmongering about dairy is overblown. In the cultures where dairy has been consumed for thousands of years, people have evolved to be able to digest it. In fact, most people with lactose intolerance can tolerate fermented dairy, like yogurt, kefir, and cheese. This is evidence that it is completely natural—or at least advantageous from an evolutionary perspective—for us to consume dairy. Dairy is also nutritious; it's packed with protein, vitamin D, potassium, phosphorus, and, of course, calcium. Grass-fed dairy, in particular, has higher concentrations of omega-3 fats, conjugated linoleic acid (CLA), and fat-soluble vitamins.[113, 114] In addition, dairy improves bone density and reduces the risk of osteoporosis.[115] Research also suggests that full-fat dairy not only does not have a harmful effect on heart disease risk, but may have a slight beneficial effect.[116] I find this research particularly fascinating because when I was in school for nutrition, which wasn't too long ago, promoting low-fat and nonfat dairy as better choices than full-fat dairy for cardiovascular disease was a given. Also, despite the claims of it being inflammatory, research suggests that dairy, especially fermented dairy, actually has a slight anti-inflammatory effect.[117]

So, if you like dairy, include it. Go for grass-fed dairy if you can afford it, and don't be afraid to go with full-fat dairy if that's what your taste buds prefer.

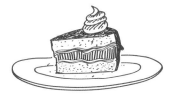

Be mindful about sweets

Now let's talk about the food that gets the gold medal for fueling the most fear and anxiety around eating: sugar.

The way sugar gets talked about makes you think it's nothing short of poison—and many people actually believe that. Whenever I hear a celebrity doctor calling sugar "poison," the image that comes to my mind is someone keeling over after eating a cookie in the same manner as Vizzini in *The Princess Bride* after drinking the glass of iocane-laced wine. Even though other health professionals don't get much training in nutrition, they should know enough about human physiology to avoid promoting such falsehoods.

So, let's take a step back and talk about what sugar is. *Sugar* is a general term used to refer to many different sweet-tasting carbohydrates that are either added to or naturally occurring in food. But even though you may be consuming sugar in different forms, your body breaks it down the same way in order to turn it into energy. To demonstrate this, here's a quick food chemistry lesson.

Table sugar is sucrose, typically extracted from sugarcane or sugar beets. It is a *di*saccharide, meaning two sugars joined together. Other disaccharides are lactose, found in dairy, and maltose, which is created when grains are broken down and fermented—in the making of beer, for example. When disaccharides are consumed, they are broken down into *mono*saccharides—glucose, fructose, and/or galactose, depending on the type of disaccharide—before being absorbed and used as energy. Now, starches and fibers are a bit more complex, as they are *poly*saccharides, which are monosaccharides and disaccharides joined together. But, like disaccharides, polysaccharides, when consumed, eventually get broken down into monosaccharides as well.

Think of monosaccharides as Lego bricks that you can join together to construct different things—in this case, various kinds of sugars, starches, and fibers. And no matter what these Lego constructions look like, when you take them apart, you end up with single Lego blocks which you can't break down any further. This is precisely what happens when you eat any kind of carbohydrate-containing foods. Because your body cannot absorb disaccharides or polysaccharides, it breaks them down to monosaccharides. And it's these monosaccharides that get absorbed into your bloodstream as an energy source.

The point of all this boring food chemistry is to show you that, despite all the fearmongering, sugar is not poison. From a biological perspective, when a monosaccharide enters your bloodstream, your cells just think of it as energy; they don't know or care where this energy came from—an apple, a cookie, some quinoa, candy, or any other source. If sugar truly was a dangerous poison, every single food that contains a speck of carbohydrate would be too.

That said, there is a kernel of truth, which is that dietary patterns high in added sugars are linked with worse health outcomes. Is this because sugar in excess is harmful, or is this because when more high-sugar foods are consumed, it means fewer nutrient-dense foods are consumed? Though my take leans more toward the latter, a little bit of both is probably true.

Much of the concern about sugar comes down to its effect on blood glucose levels. The effect of different foods on blood glucose varies widely among individuals, even for those who are not diagnosed with diabetes.[118] But in general, foods higher in added sugar and lower in fiber have a greater impact on blood sugar levels. This is especially true when a higher-sugar food is eaten by itself, as it lacks the fiber, fat, and protein that would delay gastric emptying and allow glucose to enter the bloodstream more slowly. Glucose dysregulation and persistently high blood glucose, which *can* occur from dietary patterns high in added sugar, are linked to inflammation, insulin resistance, and atherosclerosis.[119] Therefore, while individual tolerance varies, and while many people can likely eat larger quantities of sugar without it affecting their health, it's generally a smart idea to be mindful of sweets.

That said, being mindful with sweets does not mean restricting or avoiding them. Giving yourself unconditional permission with sweets is *essential* for having a good relationship with them, because, as we've discussed, restriction usually results in obsessing about that food and eating in a way that feels out of control. Instead, savor your sweets with intention and attention; tune in to the flavors and textures and let yourself fully enjoy the experience. It's also helpful to practice awareness of other aspects of the eating experience, like whether the food-policing thoughts are present or whether you are experiencing physical taste or emotional hunger—or a combination. It may feel scary to let yourself enjoy sweets, and you might fear that it will result in eating them all the time. However, research on mindful eating has shown that this actually reduces overall sweet consumption while increasing satisfaction.[120]

Myth-Busting Sugar

When it comes to sugar, misinformation abounds. Here are three of the most common myths.

MYTH: Natural sweeteners, like honey and maple syrup, are better for you.

TRUTH: Honey and maple syrup have a *slightly* lower glycemic index than table sugar, but all three are in the moderate glycemic index category.[121] Honey and maple syrup contain slightly more trace minerals and antioxidants than table sugar, but the difference is small. Nutritionally, they are just about the same. So, instead of worrying about what's better or worse from a health standpoint, consider which sweetener works best from a culinary standpoint.

MYTH: Naturally occurring sugars, like those in dairy and fruit, should be limited.

TRUTH: Even though fruit and dairy contain naturally occurring sugars, fruit contains fiber while dairy contains protein and fat, and all of these things reduce the effect of naturally occurring sugars on blood glucose levels. Also, both fruit and dairy are packed with the nutrients that research has shown to support health.

MYTH: Artificial sweeteners are healthy or unhealthy.

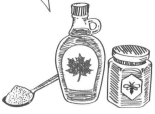

TRUTH: Depending on who you listen to, either artificial sweeteners are a healthy way to cut back on sugar or they poison your body. Much of the fearmongering is completely overblown. The claim that artificial sweeteners cause cancer has been roundly debunked.[122] And while a small study found that sweeteners may alter gut bacteria and affect blood glucose levels in some people, and some observational research has linked artificial sweeteners to diabetes, controlled studies have shown no effect.[123, 124] As for the claim that artificial sweeteners increase appetite and weight, it's not supported by most evidence.[125] All things considered, since real sugar, which we have established isn't poison, tastes much better than artificial sweeteners, I would go for the real thing.

If you're interested in learning about nutrition—and I'm guessing you are since you're reading this book—you've likely consumed a lot of literature on it and, therefore, must have come across hundreds of different tips for reducing sugar intake. These could be anything from sweetening plain yogurt with fruit to swapping sliced bananas or apples for jelly on a peanut butter sandwich, to reducing the amount of added sugar in recipes and so on. There's nothing wrong with making changes to your eating habits to reduce intake of added sugars as long as you don't feel deprived. And whether you feel deprived or not will depend on your individual food preferences. But if you do feel deprived, it's unlikely that these changes will be very helpful in the long run.

But you may be reading this and wondering how much is too much when it comes to sugar. It's impossible to say. While some organizations have put out recommendations, these are mostly based on observational studies that don't always account for other factors, like poverty and food access or how higher-sugar dietary patterns tend to be lower in other nutrients.

It's natural to desire the security of a food rule, but as you've hopefully learned, food rules aren't very helpful. In my experience, with intuitive eating, people self-moderate around sweets. By giving yourself unconditional permission, you'll stop eating sweets like it was your last chance to have them. In learning to fuel your body adequately throughout the day with satisfying meals and snacks, you'd be much less likely to need something sweet as a quick energy boost. Learning other positive coping skills also reduces emotional eating. And so overall, you'd be likely to eat sweets in a more moderate way—without trying to moderate them.

Emphasize fresh foods

Clean eating has become a popular phrase to describe eating whole, unprocessed foods. On the surface, clean eating might seem to reflect basic, healthy eating guidelines. However, it's gotten completely out of control, with most clean eating proponents pushing completely inaccurate information about innocuous food ingredients and what seems like rigid, everything-free diets. Most of the time, these clean eating diet gurus have zero training in science and nutrition, gaining their "expertise" through Google.

While it seems like each clean eating proponent has their own set of food rules, one thing they all have in common is the demonization of foods that aren't considered natural. I'm no food industry apologist, but it amazes me how the ingredients that are completely safe have been spun into some dangerous toxic chemicals just because they have difficult-to-pronounce names. I find it telling that the same gurus who warn against "unnatural" foods, made in labs and factories, are the same people who sell supplements and protein powders that are also made in labs and factories.

That said, there's a kernel of truth in what the clean eating proponents say, which is that it is good for your health to eat more fresh, whole foods. And although this is not always the case, generally speaking, fresher, minimally processed foods really are more nutrient-dense and offer more fiber, vitamins, minerals, and phytochemicals.

This, however, does *not* mean processed foods are bad; being lower in nutrition doesn't make them unhealthy. There are plenty of frozen, boxed, and canned foods that are made with lots of fresh ingredients—think of them as coming from a really big kitchen. Also, you have the freedom to eat food simply because it tastes good to you regardless of its nutrition content. We *all* have a favorite cheap convenience food, don't we? I love cheese puffs, and it doesn't matter to me that I'm not getting nutrients when I eat them. These foods are fun to eat. I know that if I'm getting balance and variety in other areas, I'm still getting adequate nutrition.

So, instead of worrying about avoiding processed foods, flip the focus to positive nutrition and consider ways to incorporate more fresh, whole foods. One of the best ways to do this is to cook at home more often, using fresh ingredients. You don't have to be a gourmet chef. If you find cooking intimidating, learn a few simple recipes and get creative by adapting them with different spices and sauces, or swapping out different types of produce.

To make cooking at home easier, don't be afraid to use convenience foods as a vehicle for more fresh foods or to save time. Things like canned beans, frozen and canned vegetables, or microwavable grains aren't very different from what you'd get if you were to cook them from fresh. It's helpful to have a variety of different sauces and dressings on hand to make simple meals—barbecue sauce for chicken, pesto to toss with roasted vegetables, or a curry sauce to simmer vegetables and proteins in, etc. Other pantry ingredients can be rounded out into a filling meal with the addition of protein and veggies. (See Chapter 6 on how to stock your kitchen.)

Pay attention to how food makes you feel

One takeaway from this book is that food and nutrition are a personal matter. While I've run through a list of general guidelines that apply to most people, how you apply them in your life will differ based on resources, food preferences, and your unique nutrition needs. Maybe one day we'll get to the point where we can find out, with perhaps a drop of blood or swab of the cheek, exactly which foods and dietary patterns are healthiest for us, but we're not there yet. Part of me hopes we never get to that point. Having all that information sounds exhausting. For now, the best thing we can do to figure out our unique nutrition needs is to pay attention to how food makes us feel.

When you become a good caretaker of your body, feeding it adequately with a wide variety of pleasurable foods, you'll begin to rebuild a trusting relationship with it. With body trust in place, there is space to notice which foods and eating patterns feel best for you. Now, I don't mean to imply that intuitive eating will give you a superhuman connection with your body. Sometimes when I say pay attention to how food makes you feel, I think people imagine intuitive eaters closing their eyes after taking a bite of food and knowing that apples are a better choice for them than pears. What I mean is that over time, and by experimenting with different foods and meals, you'll notice patterns that leave you feeling satisfied and energized with a happy digestive system.

Here are some observations from my clients:

"When I wake up early for work, my stomach feels queasy. I feel much better when I start my day with a light smoothie, then follow it up with a bigger morning snack a couple of hours later. I call it breakfast number one and breakfast number two."

"Sweet snacks like granola or protein bars make me hungry thirty minutes later. They sometimes upset my stomach too. I feel a lot better eating savory snacks, like avocado toast, cheese and crackers, or chips and dip."

"In my case, with Crohn's disease, my body is sensitive to both too much fiber and too little fiber. It's a balance that's hard to strike. Everyone says whole grains are healthier, but they tear me up for hours after eating, especially if I'm having a flare. I feel a lot better after eating white bread and pasta. I get fiber from fruits and vegetables, but they have to be cooked, otherwise they hurt my stomach also. The difference between cooked broccoli and raw broccoli is huge!"

"I've noticed I have more energy when I eat meals with more carbs and fat with just a little protein, like bean soup with avocado or creamy pasta with vegetables. Carbs feel nourishing for me, and fat makes the meal more satisfying. Whenever I have a standard meal with beef or chicken as the main dish, I feel tired."

"I sleep a lot better when I have a bigger, protein-rich breakfast and lunch and eat a light dinner."

What I appreciate about this guideline is that it's not about eating for immortality or immunity from disease; it aligns with a definition of health that includes taking care of your body in order to live life according to your values and goals and to have the space and energy to do the things you enjoy. In my professional experience, lab values and weight often scare people into making big dietary changes that aren't sustainable. When you notice how you feel after you fuel your body well, it will be a lot more motivating in the long run.

Medical Conditions, Gentle Nutrition, and Intuitive Eating

Perhaps you are reading this as someone with a health diagnosis who has been told to manage your condition with a strict diet. And you may be wondering if gentle nutrition is for you.

It's unfortunate that diet culture has infiltrated healthcare. It has resulted in people being prescribed diets much stricter than necessary when they're diagnosed with a nutrition-related health condition. With minimal training in nutrition, doctors can be just as susceptible to nutrition misinformation as anyone else. Some of my clients have been told to follow a "zero-sodium diet" for hypertension (this would kill them) or to cut out all carbohydrates for diabetes. And I have seen fad diets like intermittent fasting and keto recommended to my clients for conditions ranging from PCOS to gastric reflux to cancer— conditions in which there is next to zero evidence supporting the use of these diets.

In most cases, gentle nutrition can be used to manage health conditions. Often, it's a matter of directing the mindset toward positive nutrition and zooming out to see the big picture. For example, instead of eliminating refined grains and following a low-carb diet for diabetes, you can focus on increasing whole grains and eating consistent amounts of carbohydrate throughout the day. Instead of following a strict low-fat diet for high cholesterol, it would be smart to focus on increasing monounsaturated fats and cholesterol-lowering high-fiber foods. If you can, I encourage you to work with an intuitive eating and Health at Every Size®–aligned dietitian. Alternatively, you may be able to find intuitive eating resources for your condition online.

When considering nutrition therapy for health conditions, it's helpful to revisit the nutrition hierarchy concept. For every health condition I can think of, the bottom three tiers of the pyramid are the same. Whether you have an autoimmune condition, IBS, diabetes, or PCOS, your body still needs the same nutritional adequacy, balance, and variety as everyone else's. There may be adaptations to the top tier of the hierarchy that are health-promoting, but if the bottom three needs are not met, then these changes are unlikely to help.

That said, you get to define what gentle nutrition looks like for you. If you find through experimentation that you feel better when you eat in a way that looks more "rigid" from the outside, that's perfectly fine. Receiving a health diagnosis can be scary, and if you feel more comfortable managing it with a specific way of eating, there's nothing wrong with that. For a serious or life-altering diagnosis, you may be willing to try anything, including a strict dietary approach. It may not align with intuitive eating, but you get to decide how you want to care for and feed your body. I just hope you will be honest with yourself about the physical and mental effects and stop doing anything that isn't working for you.

If you are higher weight and have a health condition for which you have been told to lose weight, I am so sorry that you were given lazy medicine. Hopefully, by this point in the book, you know that weight is not health and that no diet has been shown to result in sustained weight loss for more than a small number of people. A doctor, dietitian, or any other healthcare provider telling you to lose weight to manage your condition is like prescribing to you a medication that works less than 5 percent of the time. So, here's something you could do: ask your provider what they would recommend for someone with a BMI of 22. More than likely, that recommendation is going to be the best approach for you too. There isn't a separate set of nutrition rules for people with bigger or smaller bodies—nutrition is nutrition!

The Healthiest Choice Isn't Always the Most Nutritious Choice

Any discussion of which food is healthiest often focuses on nutrient content—vitamins, minerals, fiber, and so on. However, nutrient content is just one aspect of making a healthy food choice; it's not all of it.

Different foods serve different purposes, and sometimes the food that's healthiest for you isn't the one that's the most nutritious. I like to use a highly exaggerated scenario to illustrate this point to my clients. Imagine driving through the desert on an empty road, when, all of a sudden, your car breaks down. With no food, water, or cell phone service, you have to walk to the next gas station, three miles away. When you finally arrive, dehydrated and dizzy with low blood sugar, what's the healthiest thing for you? A soda! It will hydrate you and quickly bring your blood sugar back up. The fact that the soda doesn't contain any fiber, antioxidants, or vitamin D doesn't matter; it's what your body needs in that moment.

It's doubtful you will ever find yourself in this situation. However, it is quite possible that you'll one day experience low blood sugar, and, when you do, whatever sweetened beverage you can find most easily will be the healthiest thing for you. Perhaps one day you will decide to run a race or compete in an intense physical activity, where a gel pack—essentially sugar with electrolytes—is a healthy choice of fuel, as it will provide your body with readily available energy. At some point in your life, you'll likely get a stomach bug, and saltines, white toast, and sodium-rich canned chicken soup will be some of the healthiest things you can eat, as they're easy to digest and will provide your body with a bit of salt to rehydrate it. And what about the time you have to wait much longer than expected to get your food at a restaurant? In that moment, a bit of white bread is the healthiest thing for you, as it brings your blood sugar up and gets some food in your stomach that also can be digested quickly so you won't be stuffed for your meal. As you can see, what's healthiest is situational and not always contingent on nutrient content.

Pleasure is also an aspect of health. You could eat all the most nutritious foods in the world, but choking them down while feeling miserable would not be not very healthy, physically or mentally. There's actually evidence indicating that enjoying your meals may help you absorb more nutrients. My favorite example is a 1970s study conducted on a group of Thai and Swedish women. It found that the Thai women absorbed more iron from a spicy, culturally appropriate dish they enjoyed, whereas the Swedish women absorbed more iron from a traditionally Swedish dish than they did from the Thai dish, which they found to be too spicy.[126] Based on what I've discussed about the effects of stress on digestion, inflammation, and overall health, can you imagine what happens when you're forcing yourself to eat something you hate three or more times a day?

Remember, health and nutrition are two different things. A food can contain more or less nutrition, but that's not the only factor that determines whether it is a healthy *choice* for you in the moment. This is why we can't label foods "healthy" or "unhealthy." Sometimes the healthiest choice is the one with the least nutrition. Nutrition is *part* of health, but it's not all of it. When you remove from yourself the pressure to eat perfectly all the time, there's room to honor other aspects of health (for example, pleasure, social connections, and having fun with food) and tune in to what makes you feel physically and emotionally satisfied at the moment. Let's not make nutrition the be-all and end-all of health or something to overcomplicate or stress over. Instead, look at nutrition as one of many tools to help you live a happier, healthier life.

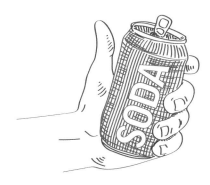

Chapter 5

MAKING CHANGES THAT LAST

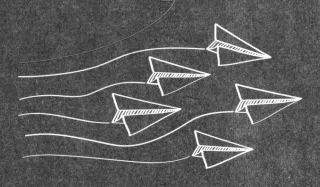

When new clients reach out to me, it's because they're ready for change. They know that what they've been doing isn't working for them. It has only made them stress and obsess over food and their bodies, and it's definitely not supporting their physical or mental health. The question they have is, "What does that change look like?"

For something we were all born with the innate ability to do, intuitive eating shouldn't be hard to adopt. But it is. It involves changing your thoughts about food, your environment, your self-care behaviors, and the types of food you eat. All of these shifts in thinking are difficult. And on top of everything lies the most difficult change of all: letting go of trying to control your body size. With dieting, you have a clear set of rules and guidelines to follow; you know exactly what that diet entails. All you have to do is pick a day on the calendar—next Monday, perhaps?—and you're ready to go.

As cliché as it sounds, intuitive eating is a journey, and it begins by taking one step. This is especially true when it comes to incorporating gentle nutrition. This chapter is not about how to start gentle nutrition because it is not a diet that you can start or stop. There are no rules, no right or wrong, and no start date. Occasionally, a client asks me something along the lines of, "So when are we going to start working on gentle nutrition?" But once they've spent some time learning what gentle nutrition really is, they come to realize that it is already a part of their eating choices in many ways. Simply by learning about intuitive eating and starting to tune in to your food, you, too, will come to realize that gentle nutrition has subconsciously influenced your food choices in one way or another.

That said, after you've done some solid work on healing your relationship with food, it can be helpful to bring in gentle nutrition in a more intentional way. Remember, there are many ways to improve health, and nutrition doesn't have to be something you give priority to. However, I hope that after having read the previous chapter, you're now finding nutrition to be more accessible than you thought.

Many people who have been practicing intuitive eating for some time are interested in learning how to feed their bodies better, but they don't want it to feel like or become a diet. This is a valid concern. So many diets have gone undercover as "lifestyle change" or "wellness" that it's hard to know sometimes where the line is between gentle nutrition and restrictive pseudo-diet.

In practice, that "line" is different for everyone because gentle nutrition looks different for everyone. What may feel gentle to one person may feel rigid to another. Gentle nutrition is all about understanding your values and intentions for pursuing health and nurturing habits that promote the behaviors that align with those values and intentions. My role as an intuitive eating counselor is to take this broad principle of gentle nutrition, break it down, and help my clients incorporate it into their lives and adapt it to their needs, taking into account their different lifestyles, skills, and barriers. I hope this chapter equips you with the tools that enable you to make the changes you find personally meaningful, both with nutrition and with other aspects of self-care.

The Biology of Why Change Is Hard

Whether you have just started your intuitive eating journey or are well along the way, I'm positive that you've often found yourself frustrated at feeling stuck in a diet mentality or trapped repeating the same behaviors around food. If it feels like intuitive eating isn't coming naturally to you, welcome to the club!

Part of the reason change is so hard is because of a neat little trick of the brain. When you repeatedly engage in a behavior, your brain creates a neural pathway, a connection between brain cells. The more often you repeat the behavior, the stronger the neural pathway becomes. This helps your brain conserve energy, especially with complex tasks. Despite being a relatively small mass of about 3 pounds or so, the brain is extremely metabolically active, representing 20 percent of the body's energy consumption.[127] Your brain is responsible for keeping your heart beating, your lungs breathing, and your temperature regulated; it controls your movement and directs pretty much every other function of your body. So, please forgive it if it takes the lazy option from time to time. Besides, these neural pathways allow you to engage in complex tasks without using a ton of mental energy. Think of how much energy it took to read a paragraph when your first learned how to read, compared to the ease with which you're able to read this paragraph right now, thanks to your neural pathways.

I like to think of these neural pathways as a well-trodden hiking trail through the woods. Years of heavy traffic have left the soil matted, solid, and free from obstruction, so the trail is pretty clear and obvious. It's a path you can walk along easily without having to pay much attention to your footing or where you are going.

Changing your thoughts and behaviors is like creating a new hiking trail of your own by cutting down brush and branches through the forest. It makes sense, therefore, that your brain would resist this energy-intensive path and want to go back to that nice and easy, well-established trail, especially when you lose sight of intentions. So, whenever you notice yourself repeating an old behavior with food, just remember how your neural pathways work and give yourself a little compassion.

That said, attempts at changing are not futile. Research in the field of neuroscience has demonstrated the brain's neuroplasticity or its ability to form new neural pathways throughout life. When we repeat a new behavior or thought pattern, the brain forms a new neural pathway, which, when reinforced, will cause the old one to lose its strength. Imagine the new hiking trail through the woods becoming easier and easier to travel as more and more pairs of feet have walked on it, while the old hiking trail gets covered with branches and brush from lack of use. This will take time, but your brain is adaptable. You can literally rewire it!

Your Intentions and Values

Before engaging with gentle nutrition, it's important to get clarity on your values and to understand your intentions. Trying to make a change without knowing about the purpose behind that change is rarely helpful or sustainable. When a goal isn't connected to your values and intentions, it will feel hollow and purposeless, making it hard for you to follow through when your energy and motivation inevitably run low. Just take a look at your to-do list and the items that keep getting bumped back another week. Those are probably the items that don't feel personally meaningful to you.

Homing in on your values and intentions will help you focus on making changes that actually improve your quality of life, rather than checking off a box of what you think you "should" do. Knowing your values and intentions provides a framework for making decisions around food and eating—a framework that helps build confidence in your ability to feed yourself competently without relying on rules and rigidity.

Intentions

An intention is a vision, a mental image of what you would like an area of your life to look like in the future, or the outcome you are expecting or hoping for in making the changes you embark on. Knowing your intentions will allow you to set priorities and use your time and headspace wisely by choosing which kinds of health behaviors you want to focus on. Non-diet intentions include managing a health condition, building strength and endurance, feeling energized and focused at work, nurturing a healthier relationship with your body, and eating more pleasurable food.

Improving health is a commonly cited intention for gentle nutrition. However, as we've discussed in Chapter 3, health is not something entirely within your control. That's not to say health is the wrong intention to set; it's just that you should think beyond a narrow definition of it. What is the purpose of pursuing health? How can it help you live a life in line with your values and other life goals?

And then there's the intention of weight loss. Whether or not you call it a diet, making a change to your eating behaviors with the goal of losing weight will trigger the diet mentality, which can sabotage your attempts at more healthful eating. Health-promoting changes, such as meal planning or eating more produce, which some diets and pseudo-diets encourage, work better when they're made without having weight loss as a goal; you're more likely to stick to them regardless of what happens to your weight.

That's not to say you need to eliminate all desire for weight loss or feel completely okay with your body before engaging with gentle nutrition. To many—if not most—people, this can feel impossible, but I encourage you to think beyond the scale in setting your intentions. Ask yourself what else you would want out of engaging in gentle nutrition if you knew it wouldn't result in weight loss. In taking the possibility of weight loss off the table, you're better able to home in on what else is important to you.

A former client of mine, Michelle, is a great example of the value of homing in on your intentions. In her seventies when we started working together, Michelle used to be quite active, especially with outdoors activities. However, after a recent injury that caused severe knee pain, she had been unable to participate in the activities she enjoyed as her knee was healing. This led to mindlessly eating large quantities of food at night out of boredom, which then led to gaining weight. Michelle, who was already in a larger body, felt extremely uncomfortable and self-conscious, especially when working out at the gym. Even after her knee had healed, she felt too uncomfortable to get back to the activities she enjoyed. When she did work out, she felt easily winded, which she blamed on her weight gain, not the fact that she had simply lost some strength and endurance from the months of inactivity as she healed. She tried dieting, thinking weight loss would help her feel more comfortable and physically able, but it just made the nighttime eating worse.

So, when Michelle first came in, her initial goal was weight loss. However, we were able to shift that focus onto an intention that was much more meaningful: getting back to the activities she enjoyed so much. We focused on eating more adequately throughout the day to help make sure Michelle's body was properly fueled for movement and for her to have more physical and mental energy to cook a satisfying dinner at night, which made her less likely to snack in front of the TV. To help with the boredom at night, Michelle started using that time to do her physical therapy exercises or go on short walks with her partner. To help her feel more comfortable in her here-and-now body, we also incorporated body image work, and identified new exercise environments in which she felt more comfortable and accepted. With these changes, Michelle was able to get back to the activities that brought her so much joy.

Looking back at Michelle's initial attempts at dieting, what's interesting is that many of the behaviors she tried to adopt during the diet attempts were actually similar to what we worked on together. She tried to eat regular meals and snacks (though carbohydrate-restricted), to do her physical therapy, to walk more often, and to cook dinner instead of snacking. But because weight loss was the intention, every time she hopped on the scale and didn't see the results she wanted, those changes would go to the wayside. Putting weight loss on the back burner gave her the headspace to engage in a real, meaningful, and lasting change.

You may be reading this and wondering if Michelle ever lost weight. To answer your question, I don't actually know. What I do know is that she feels more comfortable in her body and is having a better quality of life—all by dropping the focus on the scale.

Values

Values are the ideals and characteristics you care about. Values can describe who you want to be, what you want to do with your time on this earth, and which qualities you want to develop. Identifying your values is important because gentle nutrition doesn't lay out a strict set of rules—and neither does intuitive eating as a whole. Values serve as guiding principles for your decision-making, gently nudging you toward a way of taking care of your physical and mental health that is flexible and feels good for *you*. Values allow you to make intentional, as opposed to impulsive, choices around food and self-care. Knowing your values lets you live in the here-and-now without losing sight of the long term.

While dieting aligns with the *cultural* value of thinness, it usually doesn't align with your *individual* values for how you want to live. Not only that, but the pursuit of weight loss often runs directly against your core values. For example, if connection is a value of yours, you'll find that dieting often leads to distancing yourself from social engagements that involve food or to spending time at the gym instead of with other people. If autonomy and choice are among your values, you'll find that dieting often forces you to hand over your choices to the author of whatever plan you're following.

A client of mine, Helen, is a great example of how identifying your values can guide more health-promoting behaviors. Having struggled with chronic dieting and disordered eating for almost twenty years, Helen was in a place where she finally felt free around food. However, as an ICU nurse, Helen struggled to find time and energy to take care of her needs. Her job was intense; it took a lot out of her, often leaving her physically and emotionally drained. Ease and availability dictated Helen's food choices—understandably so. However, when we began our work together, Helen was already in a place where she finally accepted and appreciated her body, after having spent most of her life hating it. The problem was that she felt too exhausted and overwhelmed to know how to show that appreciation by treating her body more kindly.

I learned that joy, playfulness, humor, and fun were the values with which Helen most connected. Dealing with issues of life and death at work all day, she valued spending her time doing things that were more lighthearted. With that in mind, our work centered on how to make it more fun for Helen to engage in healthier behaviors.

To bring some joyful movement into her life, one idea Helen came up with was ditching her attempts to go to the gym after work, and, instead, going for post-work walks or jogs while listening to comedy podcasts and playing tennis with her sister. According to Helen, both she and her sister were awful at tennis, so it was fun for them to laugh together at their lack of skills. She also started taking movement breaks at work and got the rest of her ICU staff involved. If a few of them had some rare downtime, she'd play a fun nineties pop song, and they would have a quick dance party—a much needed mental break that I'm sure all of her coworkers appreciated.

Helen also learned that cooking could actually be fun when she gave herself a break from the expectations of cooking a full meal every night. Instead, she gave herself permission to order takeout, to have a microwave meal, or to have leftovers on the days she worked. Without the pressure, she was actually excited to cook the recipes from some food blogs that she loved and to incorporate more gentle nutrition into those recipes. As a bonus, all this home cooking often gave her the leftovers that she was excited to have on workdays as an alternative to the not-so-exciting food at the hospital cafeteria.

What Are Your Values?

Circle the values on the list below that connect with you. Try to limit the number to 10, which means you must prioritize. Is there a theme to these 10 values? How do they relate to your intentions? How can your food and self-care choices better align with your chosen values?

☐ ACCEPTANCE	☐ FAIRNESS	☐ LEADERSHIP	☐ SELF-CONFIDENCE
☐ ACHIEVEMENT	☐ FAMILY	☐ LEARNING	☐ SIMPLICITY
☐ ADVENTURE	☐ FLEXIBILITY	☐ LOVE	☐ SPIRITUALITY
☐ ADVOCACY	☐ FREEDOM	☐ LOYALTY	☐ STRUCTURE
☐ AMBITION	☐ FRIENDSHIPS	☐ MINDFULNESS	☐ SUCCESS
☐ AUTHENTICITY	☐ FRUGALITY	☐ NOVELTY	☐ TEAMWORK
☐ AUTONOMY	☐ FUN	☐ OPEN-MINDEDNESS	☐ TRADITION
☐ BALANCE	☐ GENEROSITY	☐ OPTIMISM	☐ VARIETY
☐ CALMNESS	☐ GRACE	☐ PASSION	☐ WARMTH
☐ CARING	☐ GROWTH	☐ PEACE	☐ WEALTH
☐ CHALLENGE	☐ HAPPINESS	☐ PERFORMANCE	☐ WELL-BEING
☐ COMMUNITY	☐ HEALTH	☐ PERSONAL DEVELOPMENT	☐ WISDOM
☐ COMPASSION	☐ HONESTY	☐ POWER	
☐ COMPETITION	☐ HUMOR	☐ RESILIENCE	
☐ CONNECTION	☐ INCLUSIVENESS	☐ RESOURCEFULNESS	
☐ CONSISTENCY	☐ INDEPENDENCE	☐ REST	
☐ CREATIVITY	☐ INDIVIDUALITY	☐ RISK-TAKING	
☐ CURIOSITY	☐ JOY	☐ SAFETY	
☐ DEPENDABILITY	☐ KINDNESS	☐ SECURITY	
☐ EMPATHY	☐ KNOWLEDGE		

The Power of Small Changes

The world of health and fitness glorifies big changes. Many of the popular health and fitness programs want you to mark the beginning of a "health kick" with a huge, overnight change. They tell you to go big or go home; they tell you that if it doesn't challenge you, it doesn't change you. It's no wonder many people feel that if the change they are making isn't big, it's not going to make a difference.

But big changes are rarely sustainable. Instead of teaching you to adjust to or work around things that happen in real life, like late nights at work, social events, getting sick, or stressful events, these diet and fitness challenges teach you to push through, which can work for only so long.

In psychology, the theory of *self-efficacy* describes how the belief in your ability to execute a course of action strongly determines your ability to actually carry it out. That's why it's so important to set the health goals that you feel confident in achieving in the long term.

In my professional experience, big goals that require overnight changes can be especially paralyzing for those who identify as a perfectionist. An example of this is my client Celia, with whom I worked on treating binge eating disorder. Even though Celia came to realize through our work together that her post-work binge eating was strongly related to not eating enough during the day, she couldn't seem to get into the habit of bringing adequate meals and snacks to work. Eventually, we discovered that it was perfection paralysis that was keeping her stuck. Instead of telling herself that she just needed to bring adequate amounts of food, Celia told herself that she had to bring the exact *right* foods and that each meal and snack had to be perfectly balanced. Anything less felt like a failure to her. And it was precisely this fear of failure that had kept her trapped in the same cycle.

So, together we took a step back and set a goal of picking up a few frozen meals and shelf-stable snack foods to keep at work and setting an alarm as a reminder to eat. Then we gradually worked on ways to make it easier for Celia to get adequate food in during the day, such as cooking a little extra food at dinner so she could use the leftovers to throw together easy lunches for work or ordering from the restaurants near her work that she liked. By not letting perfect be the enemy of good, she was able to get into the habit of packing lunch and taking work breaks to eat.

The little things you do make a difference; they can have a huge effect on your physical and mental health. This is true on the negative side as well: little things, like missing or not eating enough at breakfast, getting a bad night of sleep, or skipping your morning walk can affect the rest of your day. You can harness the power of small change for good by engaging in positive self-care behaviors that lead to more positive self-care behaviors. Over time, you build self-efficacy from the good feelings and the sense of accomplishment from reaching those small goals, and that confidence will help you accomplish even bigger goals and creating even bigger changes.

Healthier Habits Through Baby Steps

Creating a health-promoting habit starts with a baby step. Behavioral scientist BJ Fogg compares forming a habit to growing a plant where you find a good spot in your garden to plant a seed, then nourish it with water, sunlight, and everything else that it needs in order to grow. While the plant may need a little extra attention and care at first, eventually, the roots will get established, and all the plant needs at that point are check-ins and routine maintenance. Occasionally, there might be a disturbance to the plant's environment—a drought, for example—and it may need a bit more care and nurturing to make it through. But overall, the plant should be able to thrive without you having to put a lot of energy into it.[128]

In Fogg's analogy, the seed represents a small behavior that, hopefully, will grow into a habit. To build a habit, start by finding a good spot for a small behavior in your daily routine. For this behavior to take root and grow into a habit, you need to nurture it with positive reinforcement and celebration. Over time, once the habit has been established, it won't need much more energy to maintain, other than occasional check-ins and readjustments when some life changes come along that might disrupt it. Just as some of your initial attempts to grow a plant may fail, so may your early attempts to nurture a habit. Think of it as an opportunity for growth by taking what you learned and applying it when you try again.

Start with a tiny change

To foster a health-promoting habit, start with a baby step, a pared-down version of your desired habit. Set a goal that you feel highly confident in your ability to carry through, even when your energy and motivation run low. Remember, the larger the behavior change, the more energy and motivation it will require. You want to set yourself up for success.

Think of a messy room in your house that you want to clean. The mess can become so overwhelming that the idea of spending hours cleaning it up sounds so daunting that you don't feel like following through. What about setting a goal of cleaning and organizing one little part of the room after every workday, whether it was a desk drawer or a folder or an overflowing shelf on your bookcase? You may find that you're motivated to do a little more. Perhaps a couple of weeks later, that room will become somewhat organized, and a month later, it's all clean and tidy. Engaging in small behaviors can add up to big changes.

Below are some examples of baby steps to take to achieve large goals. How easy or difficult a behavior is will differ from person to person, so some of these examples may not resonate with you. The idea is to choose a behavior that you feel highly confident in your ability to carry through. I will continue to expand on these goals in the following section.

EAT ACCORDING TO HUNGER AND FULLNESS CUES
Check in with hunger and fullness cues once a day.

 WALK MORE
Walk around the block.

 EAT MORE VEGETABLES
Eat a vegetable.

 EAT REGULAR MEALS AND SNACKS
Eat a snack.

 MEDITATE REGULARLY
Take five deep breaths.

 DRINK MORE WATER
Drink a glass of water.

 MEAL PLAN
Plan one recipe.

 EAT MORE MINDFULLY
Eat one meal without distractions.

 SPEND MORE QUALITY TIME WITH FAMILY
Spend ten minutes quality time with family.

Find a good spot for it

For a new behavior to take root and grow into a habit, you'll want to find a good spot for it in your existing daily routine, one that can serve as a prompt or reminder to follow through with your small goal.

One study on forming a flossing habit found that the participants who were instructed to floss *after* brushing their teeth were significantly more likely to make flossing a habit than those who are instructed to floss before brushing their teeth.[129] You're more likely to follow through with a new behavior when you place it immediately after an established routine which serves as a cue. This is a method called *habit stacking*, in which you stack the desired habit on top of an established one. Another way to build a new behavior, especially one that isn't particularly pleasurable to you, is to multitask and pair it with an activity that you enjoy, like meal planning while watching a favorite reality TV show or doing physical therapy exercises while listening to a favorite podcast.

While planning in a time to do your small behavior may seem unnecessary, doing so can strengthen your intention to follow through. Research shows having a plan or an implementation intention that spells out when and, ideally, where you will complete your behavior has a moderate to large effect on whether that behavior is carried through initially and eventually automated into a habit.[130]

A 2002 study on exercise and goal-setting highlights how having a plan is much more effective than motivation alone.[131] In the study, participants were divided into three groups: a control, a group that received a motivational presentation on the benefits of physical activity, and a group that received the same motivational presentation and were also asked to create a goal for when and where they would participate in at least twenty minutes of activity each week. The group that created a plan was more than twice as likely to exercise at least once a week compared to the other two groups. Furthermore, the group that received only the motivational presentation exercised at the same rate as the control group, showing that motivation alone is rarely enough to promote change.

Here are some ideas for how to find a good spot, using the examples of small behaviors from the previous section.

EAT ACCORDING TO HUNGER AND FULLNESS CUES
Check in with hunger and fullness cues after plating your dinner.

WALK MORE
Walk around the block after coming home from work.

EAT MORE VEGETABLES
Eat a vegetable with your favorite lunch food.

EAT REGULAR MEALS AND SNACKS
Eat a snack with an afternoon work break.

MEDITATE REGULARLY
Take five deep breaths after brewing coffee.

DRINK MORE WATER
Drink a glass of water after brushing your teeth in the morning.

MEAL PLAN
Plan one recipe while watching your favorite Sunday morning TV show.

EAT MORE MINDFULLY
Turn off the TV after you finish cooking dinner.

SPEND MORE QUALITY TIME WITH FAMILY
Spend ten minutes of quality time with family after you finish eating dinner.

Before trying to start a new habit, pause to make sure you have the resources you need. In gardening, you'd make sure all the gardening equipment is in place before planting a seed; likewise, in building a new habit, you want to be prepared with the resources you need to carry out that change. Ask yourself what you absolutely need, what would be helpful, and how you can create an environment that is conducive to your habit.

For example, if your goal is to eat more whole grains, you absolutely need actual whole grains to be available for you to eat. A few simple and tasty recipes that incorporate whole grains would be helpful in this case. Lastly, to create an environment that's conducive to eating more whole grains would be to stock up your kitchen with whole-grain items that require little to no preparation, like whole-grain bread, microwave-ready or frozen brown rice, or whole-grain crackers.

Nourish your habit

Just as a plant needs water and sunlight, your habit will need nourishment too, but in the form of positive reinforcement and celebration of success.

And this is one of the reasons dieting can be so seductive. The scale offers a huge positive reinforcement—at least, while the diet is "working." Add to that the compliments and positive feedback from others. You can see why people keep going back to it even after dozens of failed attempts in the past.

For most people, it's probably not realistic to conjure the same amount of positive emotion you get for checking in with hunger and fullness as you get with weight loss. However, that doesn't mean you shouldn't celebrate those little steps. Celebrating your successes and letting yourself feel positive emotions may seem silly and unnecessary, but this is important.

The broaden-and-build theory of psychology explains how positive emotions foster expanded thinking, creativity, and resilience to adversity.[132] This theory has been applied to the science of behavior change, creating what's called an *upward spiral of lifestyle change.* This is when the positive emotions felt during and after the behavior motivate further engagement with and expansion of the behavior and build psychological, social, and physical resources to continue engaging in the behavior.[133] Barbara Fredrickson, the psychologist who developed the broaden-and-build theory states, "Positive emotions achieve what New Year's resolutions cannot by motivating sustained adherence to health behaviors by the carrot of flexible, nonconscious desire, rather than the whip of rigid, conscious willpower."[134] Giving yourself a pat on the back for eating a piece of fruit at breakfast might seem pretty lame, but that positive emotion will help cement your behavior, expand upon it, and build skills for continuing the behavior through the challenges that inevitably arise.

While positive emotions expand thinking, negative emotions, like anxiety, fear, and failure, have been shown to narrow thinking.[135] With negative emotions, you're more likely to miss the forest for the trees. You can see how experiencing shame and failure after making a perceived mistake harms one's ability to change in the long term. These negative emotions trigger a fight-or-flight effect in the brain, which chips away at your ability to solve problems creatively.

Resilience

Change is incredibly hard, and moments of failure are inevitable. Not only that, life also happens, and even when a behavior has become a habit, things can happen to throw your routine off course. Failure provides an opportunity for learning and growth, and it can sometimes be a humbling reminder that the goal you've set isn't very realistic. But in order to learn from failures or mistakes, you've got to have the resilience to look at what happened in a nonjudgmental way and to not blame yourself.

A client of mine, Keith, is an example of resilience through failures. Having grown up in a low-income family, Keith worked multiple jobs from the time he was fourteen to pay his way through college. Because of that, he was used to being on the go and fending for himself with food—fast food. But now in his thirties, Keith was ready to learn basic self-care with food, especially after a gallbladder surgery that left him sensitive to higher-fat foods.

Keith set a goal to cook more nutritious meals at home, but he couldn't seem to be able to make it happen. Though hard on himself at times, Keith learned from multiple failed attempts that cooking on a work night just wasn't going to happen, that trying to cook a new recipe was much too intimidating, and that he needed to clean out his overflowing and overwhelming pantry because it stressed him out too much when he tried to cook. Eventually, we figured out that by preparing dishes that Keith was already familiar with (and looking for ways to add nutrients with whole grains and more produce), he became more comfortable in the kitchen and cooked more often. Keith still eats fast food with unconditional permission when he's in the mood for it or when he doesn't have time to cook, but preparing pleasurable, nutritious meals has become a habit for him.

Another aspect of resilience is being able to adapt to disruptions to your usual routine and to recognize the need to recalibrate. It is also very normal to go through seasons of life where nutrition or other health-promoting behaviors take a back seat for one reason or another. After all, when it comes to health, what matters is the big picture, not the day-to-day.

One of my clients, Brianna, regularly went through periods where her usual health habits had to take a back seat. She was in her residency, and her hours could shift dramatically from week to week. When we started working together, Brianna was so burnt out from pseudo-dieting, trying to pack all of her meals and snacks and to work out regularly, that she had spent the past few months eating vending-machine and cafeteria foods at the hospital and takeout or frozen pizzas at home. At the same time, she could never work up the energy to exercise.

Instead of having Brianna focus on how to eat better and move more when she was in a hectic rotation, I encouraged her to accept the season of life that she was in and to just focus on getting through it. Lowering expectations of yourself is a hard pill to swallow for a smart and accomplished young doctor, but Brianna understood how her perfectionism was getting in the way. With more headspace and less shame over not meeting her goals, she was able to focus on creating health-promoting habits in rotations where she *did* have time by learning easy and satisfying meals she could make, occasionally going to the classes she enjoyed, working in mental self-care with meditation and restorative yoga, and catching up on sleep. As a perfect example of the upward spiral of lifestyle change, Brianna noticed that some of these behaviors even carried over to when she was in a hectic rotation, like packing satisfying snacks and doing restorative yoga after work. Accepting that you're in a season of life where self-care behaviors may take a back seat reduces shame and creates space for these behaviors to come back in when you're out of that season.

Self-Compassion

As you intentionally work on intuitive eating and gentle nutrition, you're bound to have moments where you don't feel so great about your eating behaviors. Whether it's blowing past fullness and feeling stuffed, flirting with pseudo-dieting, or making an impulsive food choice that leaves you feeling *bleh,* mistakes with food are bound to happen. It's important to be able to learn and move on.

Approaching those mistakes with self-criticism and shame is more likely to get you trapped in a cycle of repeating them. Self-compassion is the antidote, pulling you out of the shame cycle and giving you the headspace to build the skills needed to make different choices in the future. Self-compassion is a skill that increases health-promoting behaviors, with research linking it to improvement in sleep behaviors, eating habits, movement, and stress management.[136] Going back to the broaden-and-build theory, remember how negative emotions trigger a fight-or-flight response and narrowed thinking? That's not exactly helpful for promoting change. On the contrary, approaching your mistakes with interest and curiosity will open up room for you to be more creative in solving problems.

Here's a self-compassion exercise to help you reverse the shame and turn it into a learning experience.

First, think back to when you made an eating choice that you regretted. Remove yourself from the situation by pretending it happened to someone you care about. We are so much more understanding with other people, so getting this distance can be helpful in fostering self-compassion. Now, imagine that person you love explaining to you their eating mistake and what led up to it.

Next, neutrally evaluate the situation and try to figure out the cause. Pretend you're a scientist trying to come up with a hypothesis. Could it be stress? Extreme hunger? Fatigue? Something else?

Finally, ask yourself if there's anything that person could have done differently. Are there resources that might have been helpful? Is there some kind of self-care that they might have needed? Could the mistake have been prevented by eating adequately throughout the day or by choosing more pleasurable food? Could the backlash eating have been triggered by a physical or emotional restriction around food?

Running through this exercise helps you take away the shame, be compassionate to yourself, come up with a neutral—and likely accurate—explanation for what happened, and be equipped with useful information for when a similar situation inevitably arises again.

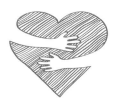

Self-Care

As discussed in Chapter 3, health is much more than nutrition. When it comes to individual behaviors that impact health, we have to look beyond food. After all, food and eating decisions don't occur in a bubble; how you eat is affected by sleep, stress, physical activity, and other variables. This section discusses tips and strategies for making changes in other aspects of self-care, including sleep, stress management, and movement.

Sleep

While sleep is a time for rest, it's also a time for your brain to get to work, organizing memories, repairing tissue, growing muscle, and synthesizing hormones. When you get enough sleep, your brain has better decision-making ability, concentration, memory, and reaction time. You feel more alert and energized, and your hunger and fullness cues are better regulated. I could go on about the benefits of adequate sleep, but I think we've all had personal experiences with a lack of sleep that have shown us just how important sleep is.

THE NATIONAL SLEEP FOUNDATION'S RECOMMENDATIONS FOR SLEEP[145]

Age Group	Recommended Sleep Per Day
Teen (13–18)	8–10 hours
Adults (18–65)	8–9 hours
Older Adults (65+)	7–8 hours

Sometimes a lack of sleep is a choice, like when you stay up late watching TV or wake up very early for work or exercise. Other times, there are medical and psychological reasons for it, like anxiety, insomnia, sleep apnea, or medications that interfere with sleep. While the former may be an easier fix, both can be improved with good sleep habits.

Certain activities relax you and help you fall asleep. Reading (or listening to) bedtime stories often does the trick. My favorite way to fall asleep is to recall a happy and relaxing vacation memory, starting at the very beginning and walking myself through it, recalling and lingering on cozy little details.

Sometimes a bedtime snack helps. Try a food with carbs paired with fat and/or protein, such as a small bowl of cereal and milk or ice cream, or a handful of crackers with peanut butter or trail mix. Diet culture spreads a lot of fear around eating at night, but nothing will keep you tossing and turning like going to bed on an empty stomach. In addition, be sure to eat regular meals and snacks during the day. The circadian rhythm, our twenty-four-hour sleep-wake cycle, is impacted not only by light and dark but by meal timing as well.[137]

Establishing a regular bedtime can also be helpful. This helps establish a flow to your day, which can help you fall asleep faster. It's also helpful to create a comfortable sleep environment: a calm, relaxing, clean, and uncluttered bedroom that's dark and cool, ideally

65°F to 67°F; temperature seems to be one of the most important factors impacting sleep.[138] Be sure to limit blue light, whether it's from the sun, your TV, or scrolling on your cell phone in bed, as blue light impacts melatonin levels, disrupting both quantity and quality of sleep.[139] Instead, keep a journal by your bed so you can unload troubling thoughts or brain-dump tomorrow's tasks in order to go to sleep with a clearer mind.

In addition, research shows that regular physical activity is helpful for both sleep quality and quantity.[140] I often recommend that my clients try yoga, especially restorative yoga, prior to going to bed as part of a calming bedtime routine. It can help with sleep as well as anxiety, depression, and mood.[141]

Lastly, remember that caffeine and alcohol play a part in the quality of your sleep. Caffeinated beverages consumed after the mid-afternoon can disrupt sleep. Alcohol has also been shown to negatively affect sleep at all dosages, although higher quantities have a more significant detrimental effect on sleep length and quality.[142] If you're struggling with sleep, it might be smart to be mindful of how much alcohol you consume, especially on weeknights.

Stress Management

It is impossible to address nutrition without discussing stress management. Stress has a huge impact on food choices. When your brain is overwhelmed with stress, you're likely to default to old, familiar behaviors. Sometimes that's okay—after a stressful day, perhaps thinking about gentle nutrition takes more mental energy than you've got. Think about how there will be more meals and snacks in the future. Remind yourself that eating a dinner of cheese crackers while curled up in the fetal position on the couch is not going to make or break your health. However, when stress is chronic, these default behaviors can add up and create additional stress by zapping your body of the energy that good nutrition can supply.

Research has shown that meditation helps with stress management and health conditions. It can help lower many of the biological side effects of acute stress, like stress hormones and heart rate.[143] Turning a stroll outside into a mindful walk is also beneficial. As you walk, involve all your senses. Notice the fresh air, how your feet feel when they touch the ground, the sounds around you, and the little details you see on your walk. Pretend you're a photographer and mentally capture pretty little details like the brick patterns on a house, flowers in bloom, or puffy clouds in the sky.

Having someone to talk to helps as well. Emotional support is important in combating stress. Create a list of people in your life whom you trust. Next to each name, make a list of topics you feel comfortable talking to them about. Consider regular therapy, which should seem as normal as going to the doctor for your yearly physical. We all need and deserve a safe space to process emotions, talk through struggles, and explore possible solutions.

The stress management aspect of self-care doesn't need to be all about what people think of as boring preventative maintenance, like taking your medications, going to therapy, or setting boundaries at work. You can try to practice what I call "fluffy self-care": i.e., little ways of pampering yourself, like getting a manicure, treating yourself to a massage, shopping, or going out for fancy coffee. Sometimes the best self-care is cutting something out that's causing you stress. This could be a constant connection to your phone, a toxic relationship, or a voluntary commitment you don't have the time or the headspace for.

Movement

Movement for pleasure is one of the principles of intuitive eating, and when it comes to the upward spiral of lifestyle change, I find it to be particularly relevant. There's something about moving your body for fun that fuels more health-promoting behaviors and acts of self-care.

However, if you've ever used exercise as a form of weight control, setting goals around movement can be challenging because even small things like taking the stairs or going for a walk can get caught up in dieting and feel like a punishment or a form of restriction. You deserve to move your body without trying to manipulate it and to challenge your body without trying to change it. Bringing pleasurable physical activity into your life is a powerful tool for managing stress and an act of body kindness.

Sometimes the best place to start when you want to engage in regular physical activity in a sustainable way is to take a break from your regular physical activity. This sounds counterintuitive, but if you're stuck in a cycle of overexercising and burning out, just pause for a while. Wait until you feel a desire to move your body. When you do, start slowly and pay attention to what you find enjoyable.

Respect your ability and recognize that your body is built differently from other people's. That's not a good or a bad thing; it just is. Your body may be less able to do certain activities due to injury or a chronic condition. Activities that may be accessible to others may not be readily accessible to you, and that's okay. You deserve to engage with movement in a way that feels comfortable, pleasurable, and safe for you.

If you're just beginning to get more active, remember to start small. Stop setting goals where you're immediately going from zero to five days a week of cardio and strength training at the gym. Explore different types of movement to see what you enjoy. Remember, the idea is to do something that fosters positive emotions so that you actually *want* to engage in movement. Don't try to force yourself into an exercise goal that feels soul-sucking and exhausting.

Research shows that accruing physical activity in bouts of less than ten minutes is just as beneficial to health as longer sessions; in fact, it may be even more beneficial to cardiovascular health.[144] What I love about this research is that it shows the benefits of being intuitive with movement. When you feel a desire to move, you can step outside and walk around the block, throw on a song or two and dance, or practice a few minutes of yoga between meetings. There's no need to commit to anything longer if you're not in the mood or if it's not accessible to you at the time. You can even turn movement into a social activity to help redirect the focus from calorie-burning to relationship-building. Consider activities that you can do with other people, like hiking, tennis, or roller-skating, or plan a date to take a fitness class together.

Diet Mentality in Gentle Nutrition

Dieting steals time, energy, and headspace. It can also rob you of your ability to make meaningful, health-promoting changes in your life. By turning vegetables into health food, movement into a chore, and your body into a problem, dieting creates an intense pressure that's bound to trigger backlash and rebellion.

Don't let diet mentality steal your ability to engage with intuitive eating and gentle nutrition. It's all too easy for it to sneak into what's supposed to be a flexible practice and to try to impose rigid rules on you. Reclaim your ability to pursue health by challenging the all-or-nothing mindset. One of the most powerful phrases you can say in intuitive eating is "most of the time" or even "some of the time." Challenge the part of you that wants rigid rules to confirm you're "doing it right."

As you begin to disentangle diet mentality from health-promoting behaviors, keep in mind that a behavior on its own doesn't determine whether it's gentle nutrition or a diet. You could do strength-building exercises to feel strong and prevent injury or in an attempt to lose weight and tone. You could eat more vegetables to aid digestion or as a way of controlling portions of other foods you fear. In both examples, the former is intuitive eating; the latter is a pseudo-diet.

That said, if engaging with gentle nutrition were contingent on totally ridding yourself of the diet mentality, hardly anyone would be able to practice it. While we want to beware of diet mentality sneaking its way in, it's also important to recognize that it is *highly* likely to happen in one way or another. Well-known body image therapist Ashlee Bennett stated on the intuitive eating podcast *Don't Salt My Game*, "We live in a world where we're constantly immersed in diet culture. Expecting not to take any of that in is like expecting a fish not to take in any water."[145] I agree with that statement, and that's why I don't think it's reasonable to expect diet mentality to never again play a role in your decisions around food, as it very likely will. So, don't feel like you need to hold off on engaging with gentle nutrition until you have eliminated every last speck of diet mentality from your brain. And when diet mentality worms its way back in from time to time, please know that you haven't failed at intuitive eating.

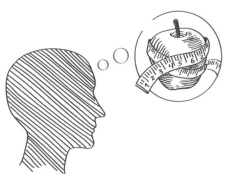

Chapter 6
MEAL PLANNING FOR SATISFACTION

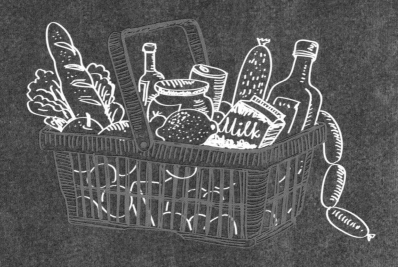

Honoring hunger by fueling your body adequately is an essential element of intuitive eating. A well-nourished body and brain will open up its other principles to you, providing you with the headspace to make intentional, as opposed to impulsive, decisions around food. One of the main goals of intuitive eating is to help you think and stress less about eating, and that goal is impossible to reach when your hungry brain is intensely focused on food.

Diet culture has created an environment that's left most people completely disconnected from what it looks like to eat a nutritious and satisfying meal. In my twelve years of practice as a dietitian, I've seen our culture cycle through countless diets. We are exposed to so many mixed messages about what and how much to eat that it's no wonder most people feel completely lost over how to eat normally.

And because we're humans, not only do we learn from observing others, but, as demonstrated by the application of social comparison theory to eating behaviors, we also have a tendency to make so-called upward comparisons wherein we compare ourselves to those we perceive as superior to us and seek to mimic them.[146] It's unfortunate that there aren't many intuitive eating role models around and that we're left with the wellness influencers, celebrities, and people whose bodies we idolize dictating the way we eat. Those struggling with body image, having a history of disordered eating, or having grown up without structure or security with food are the most vulnerable when it comes to food choices and are the most likely to fall prey to diet culture.

This can happen even within the circle of gentle nutrition. Unfortunately, as body positivity and intuitive eating have grown in popularity, more and more wellness influencers and fitness gurus, who haven't done the work themselves, are hopping on the bandwagon.

Comparing yourself to these not-so-healthy role models creates stress and confusion and further disconnects you from your body's needs. Comparing your plate to others' or what you eat to what you perceive others to be eating leads to an eating pattern that's rooted in the desire to mimic those people's behaviors instead of listening to your own body.[147] Rather than look inward, you look outward to people who are likely just as confused about food as you are. And even if they truly are experts on food, it still doesn't mean they are experts on you, your body, or your needs.

Instead of directing your attention to these outside influences, intuitive eating calls on you to honor hunger and fullness as well as your physical and emotional needs with food. But when you've lived your life totally disconnected from these internal cues, something seemingly as simple as deciding what to eat can feel overwhelming. To the people who fit this description, being told to eat according to hunger cues and what sounds satisfying in the moment is akin to being asked to read a foreign language. Many of my clients don't even know which foods they like!

If you aren't quite sure where to start, consider this chapter a primer on how to fuel your body. The tools provided in this chapter will ensure that you are meeting the bottom two tiers of the Nutrition Hierarchy of Needs discussed in Chapter 4 and will make it easier for you to meet the third tier. It covers the basics of meal planning and provides a flexible structure for preparing a balanced and satisfying meal.

Because gentle nutrition requires some advance thought in order to ensure easy access to nutritious and tasty foods, this chapter also covers how to stock your kitchen. The goal is to prevent last-minute scrambling when you're ravenously hungry, which often precipitates impulsive eating. It's my hope that this chapter will help you think about meal planning in a way that is more constructive and centers on self-care.

Fullness Versus Satisfaction

As you're learning about the tools that will help you plan satisfying meals in this chapter, I think it's important to clarify the difference between *satisfaction* and *fullness*. These two words are often used interchangeably, but there is a very important difference between them.

Fullness is the *physical* sensation of satiety, whereas satisfaction is the *mental* sensation of satiety. It's possible to feel full after eating without feeling satisfied. If you've ever eaten to the point where you're physically full but still wanted to continue eating in search of satisfaction, then you have likely experienced this. This is because we all eat for reasons other than energy and fuel. Research has shown that while feeling full is *part* of satisfaction, what plays a greater role is the sensory experience of eating.[148] As humans, we are hardwired to seek out pleasure from food through this sensory experience. Without satisfaction, therefore, it's unlikely you'll turn off the drive to eat.

One of the many reasons diets don't work is precisely because they often emphasize fullness over satisfaction. Think of some calorie-restricted diets that allow you to eat fruits and vegetables to your heart's content but little else, low-carb diets with absurd amounts of protein, or all those diet tips that tell you to drink a large glass of water or have a bowl of brothy soup before meals. Filling up on these voluminous foods may make you feel *physically* full on fewer calories, but in the long run, the lack of satisfaction will only set you up for overeating or bingeing later on.

On the other hand, it's possible also for foods to be satisfying but not filling; candy, desserts, and many snack foods, like chips, fall into this category. These foods are helpful for satisfying taste hunger, but when consumed by themselves, they would have to be consumed in large, tummy ache–inducing quantities in order for you to feel full—and that feeling of fullness most likely will not last long.

This chapter gives you some tools to help you achieve *both* physical fullness and mental satisfaction from eating. That said, the goal is not for you to feel like you need to leave every single meal and snack feeling 100 percent full and satisfied. Sometimes you miss the mark and don't eat enough; other times you may not have access to pleasurable foods, or a meal you've prepared or ordered doesn't turn out as expected. All of this is okay. The beauty of intuitive eating is that when you're giving yourself unconditional permission around food, you can move on with life knowing that more pleasurable food will be available in the future.

Planning Satisfying Meals

To feel fueled, energized, and relaxed around food, your body needs satisfying meals that both provide enough energy and are pleasurable to eat. However, what feels satisfying to you and the amount that fuels you sufficiently will change from day to day. And while you may know what foods are generally pleasurable to eat, the foods you're in the mood for will also change from day to day. This is where intuitive eating skills help you decide how much and what types of food to eat in order for you to feel satisfied.

However, when you're first trying to build intuitive eating skills, you may not have the internal cues to draw from when deciding what to eat. You know you can't trust external food rules, and you don't want to fall into pseudo-dieting; at the same time, you feel like you can't trust your body to make intuitive decisions around food either. So, you end up trying to make a decision about what to eat without reliable information. This makes food choices so much more stressful than they need to be, when the reason you got interested in intuitive eating in the first place is to stress less about food.

Also, we don't live in a world where it's always possible to make food choices on the fly. Sometimes life provides space for purely spontaneous and in-the-moment food choices; often, however, commitments to work, family, friends, and community demand otherwise. Whether it's packing a lunch for work or deciding what to buy at the store, it's helpful to have some guidance for meal planning that isn't rooted in restriction.

This is why understanding how to plan satisfying meals can be helpful. To help my clients stress less about food choices, I introduce them to a flexible tool for planning satisfying meals that I call "The Gang." I stole the term from a dear friend and fellow non-diet dietitian Kylie Mitchell, who, when creating a meal that contains all of the components for satisfaction proclaims, "The gang is all here!" The Gang is essentially a checklist you can run through to make sure your meal has what it needs for satisfaction. When The Gang is present on your plate, you're more likely to leave that meal feeling satisfied and adequately fed. When you don't have the whole gang on your plate, it's not wrong per se, but you probably won't feel as satisfied as you would if all of them were present. And because the meal likely won't turn off the drive to eat, you may continue to think or obsess about food, feel hungry again soon after, or just keep eating in hopes of finding satisfaction.

THE GANG

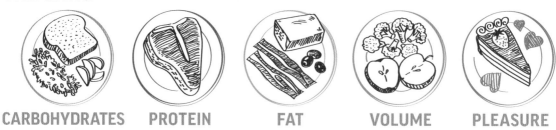

CARBOHYDRATES   PROTEIN   FAT   VOLUME   PLEASURE

The Leader of the Pack: Carbohydrates

 Thanks to diet culture, carbs are often thought of as optional. In reality, however, they are essential for making you full, satisfied, and adequately fueled from what you eat. Glucose from carbohydrates is the body's main source of energy.[149] The current dietary guidelines recommend that approximately 45 to 65 percent of energy comes from carbohydrates.[150] Carbs are used by every cell in the body. In addition, they are the *only* source of fuel that the brain can use. Remember, the brain uses about 20 percent of the body's energy, so your body has a high demand for carbohydrates, even when it is at rest. For this reason, your body has built-in systems to ensure it's getting enough carbohydrate, and it lets you know, through intense hunger, anxiety, and food obsessions, when it's not. Just think about how you feel when your blood sugar is low: dizzy, shaky, fatigued, and very ready to demolish a box of cookies. You don't get similar signals when your body has low levels of amino acids or fatty acids in the blood, and this is a clue as to just how important carbohydrates are.

When you eat a food containing carbohydrate, your body breaks it down into glucose during digestion. That glucose is absorbed from the small intestine into the bloodstream. Your hypothalamus knows *exactly* how much energy and carbohydrate you need, and it couldn't care less about any weight loss goals you may have. The hypothalamus is able to get a sense of your total body supply of glucose available for both short-term use and long-term storage, and it gets nervous when short-term glucose supply is running low. When glucose from carbohydrates enters the bloodstream, the hypothalamus detects that rise, calms down a bit, and reduces hunger hormones while sending out fullness hormones as a signal to stop eating.

Generally speaking, the amount of glucose that you get from an adequate meal will last three to four hours before your blood sugar starts to dip again. Toward the end of this range, your body has worked through glucose provided in that meal. Because most of the food empties from your stomach in two to five hours and is out of the small bowel (where glucose absorption takes place) in two to six hours, there's no more carbohydrate from food for the body to pull glucose from.[151]

While three to four hours is a general guideline for eating frequency, this is highly variable. An active young person needs more frequent refuels, whereas an older person who works a desk job might be able to go longer on a single tank. Activity levels also affect how long a meal or snack lasts, along with other factors like stress levels, sleep, and time of the month for those who ovulate. This is why listening to hunger and fullness cues is so essential.

It is possible to eat a meal that fills you up without carbohydrate. On a high-fat and high-protein diet, you can fill up on a giant steak and side salad or an omelet with veggies and cheese. But while you can fool your stomach, you can't fool the hypothalamus. Your hypothalamus knows what your body needs, and it will fight for adequate fuel. Skipping out on carbs may work for you in the short term, but, more likely, it would make you daydream about bagels and pasta and set you up for overeating or bingeing. So, instead of fighting biology, recognize the importance of carbohydrate and plan to eat sources of it at most, if not all, of your meals.

This is also a good place for me to bring up an aspect of gentle nutrition that highlights the benefits of whole grains and other high-fiber carbohydrate sources. Compared to refined grains, whole grains leave the stomach more slowly, keeping your blood sugar levels stabilized for a longer period of time.[152] There's nothing wrong, however, with white bread, white rice, or refined pasta, which, when paired with fat, protein, and produce, will leave you more than satisfied. But fiber-rich carbs like whole-grain bread and pasta, brown rice, quinoa, oats, potatoes, and beans may be more helpful for keeping you comfortable until the next time you eat.

There may be times when you intentionally or unintentionally go a longer period without eating carbohydrates. Thankfully, we have a backup supply of glucose in the liver, so as long as that's available, you won't keel over from low blood sugar. However, this is when your brain will send out cues to eat and when you will start to feel the effects of the dipping levels of glucose. You can try to suppress those feelings, or you can just eat.

Also, eating carbohydrates regularly spares the body from utilizing protein as a fuel source. This helps preserve your muscle mass, strength, and mobility through life. Just because you can survive eating less carbohydrate doesn't mean that you'll thrive. So, instead of pushing yourself to go as long as possible without eating and feeling like junk in the process, just eat!

Sidekick #1: Protein

 Protein-containing food is another member of The Gang to include as part of your meals. You probably already know that protein is important: diet culture has made us believe protein has an almost mythical health-promoting status and pushes on us massive quantities of it in the name of weight loss, muscle building, and satiety. No wonder most people are fearful of eating too much fat or carbohydrate but have no such anxiety around protein.

As with many beliefs in the world of nutrition, this one contains a kernel of truth, which is that protein plays a crucial role in promoting satiety. When you eat protein, your body breaks it down into amino acids, which are then absorbed into the bloodstream. As the level of amino acids in the blood rises, the hypothalamus releases the hormones that signal you to stop eating. Compared to fat and carbohydrate, protein promotes the greatest release of peptide YY, a hormone that reduces appetite, and also decreases levels of ghrelin, a hormone that stimulates appetite.[153, 154] You can see why protein is an important member of The Gang.

That said, protein isn't as magical as it's made out to be. Let's leave room on the plate for other enjoyable foods. Remember, we know from research on longevity that more plant-centered dietary patterns are associated with health. So, even though eating a massive chunk of chicken at lunch might mean that you can make it longer without a snack, it doesn't necessarily mean that it's health-promoting. When it comes to planning a satisfying meal or choosing a meal in a situation where you might have to go a while before eating again, knowing about protein's effect on satiety helps you take advantage of it. But there's no need to load up on huge quantities of protein at every meal.

Some people equate a satisfying meal with a meal containing a larger amount of protein, and though there's nothing wrong with that, there is only so much protein that your body can use. Even though it varies from person to person, research suggests that the maximum of protein your body can use per meal is about 0.4 gram for each kilogram of your body weight. That's about 30 to 35 grams for a 170-pound woman or a 200-pound man; this translates to a palm-sized piece of chicken. When you eat more protein than your tissues need, the excess gets broken down; part of it is excreted through your urine, and other parts are stored away in fat tissue. And don't forget that meat isn't the only protein source for your meal; other foods on your plate can provide small amounts of protein.

By engaging curiosity in intuitive eating, you may notice over time that different quantities or types of protein feel good for you in different situations. For example, a higher-protein lunch may help stave off an afternoon slump, while a simple scoop of nut butter in your oatmeal may be enough protein to satisfy you at breakfast. Regardless, I encourage you to include at least one food on your plate that is a significant source of protein.

Sidekick #2: Fat

 Along with carbohydrates and protein, your body requires fat for a satisfying meal. Fat equals fullness. When you eat a meal that contains fat, the sensors in your small intestine detect the higher-fat contents leaving your stomach.

In response, your body tries to keep food in your stomach longer by releasing hormones that slow gastric emptying. This is helpful both for stabilizing your blood glucose levels (because the carbs from your meal will also leave your stomach more slowly) and for keeping you full longer. Cholecystokinin, a hormone that stimulates the digestion of fat and protein, also alerts the hypothalamus to signal satiety, similar to how the hypothalamus detects rising blood glucose after a meal and turns off hunger cues in response.

Fat also makes food taste better and, therefore, emotionally satisfying. Fat enhances flavor by dissolving and concentrating the flavor components of food, which can then be detected by the taste receptors in the nose.[155] In cooking, fat creates certain textures and mouthfeels. It can make foods crisp and crunchy; it can also provide creaminess. Fat seems to provoke a particular pleasure response by increasing levels of dopamine, a pleasure hormone, and serotonin, a happy hormone.[156] This explains why human beings have an innate preference for high-fat foods; it makes sense from an evolutionary perspective because fat is energy-dense and a valuable source of nutrition, so we'd be highly motivated to seek it out.

As I've reiterated throughout this book, human beings are flexible, and there's no exact amount of fat you need to include as part of your meals. There is no need to intentionally cram fat into your meals, but there's no need to skimp on it either. Some meals will be higher in fat than others, and that's okay. As a general guideline, I usually recommend including at least one or two sources of fat in each meal.

The Generous Friend: Volume

 Not only does the body want all of the macronutrients for a satisfying meal, but it also wants enough volume of food to feel full. This is because along with the mechanisms that sense the presence of fat, protein, and carbohydrate, the stomach has stretch receptors that are triggered as it fills.

How much food you need to feel full and energized isn't static. However, with intuitive eating, you'll come to notice the general amounts that feel good for you. This is a place where the hunger and fullness scale in Chapter 2 comes in handy. It can help you determine a stopping point where you've had enough to eat without veering into uncomfortably full territory. For the most part, you'll want to feel a slight roundness or full sensation in your stomach without feeling physical discomfort.

Fruits and vegetables can be helpful in triggering those stretch receptors and promoting fullness. Produce is more voluminous, with a high water content. In addition to being rich in vitamins, minerals, and phytochemicals, fruits and vegetables also contain fiber, which provides bulk and keeps you fuller longer. Although you can certainly have a satisfying meal without a fruit or vegetable, for both gentle nutrition and satiety, it's smart to aim to include produce with most of your meals.

With its obsessive focus on minimizing every last calorie, diet culture often focuses on vegetables over fruits, overlooking the fact that the difference between the calorie counts of fruits and those of vegetables aren't that great—a 60-calorie difference between an apple and a cup of broccoli, for example. Both fruits and vegetables are rich in nutrients, packed with fiber, and filling. I say, go with what you enjoy and what makes sense in your meal. When you focus on eating produce in the ways that you *enjoy*, you're likely to eat more produce in general.

The Fun Friend: Pleasure

Last, but certainly not least, is pleasure. Personally, I think pleasure is the most important part of your plate. Feeding your body is a powerful act of self-care, one that, hopefully, you are engaging in multiple times a day.

So far, I have discussed the biological triggers for fullness. However, we're also aiming for satisfaction here, and that means including a serving of pleasure on your plate. Eating for satisfaction is the core of intuitive eating, yet pleasure is often overlooked in the drive to eat the "perfect" diet. Many people fear that if they allow themselves to eat the foods that they find pleasurable, they won't be able to stop eating. In my experience, when you're giving yourself unconditional permission with food, the opposite is true. We are driven to seek out pleasure from food.

It might feel uncomfortable to prioritize pleasure. Here in America, food is often feared. Psychologist Paul Rozin has studied attitudes toward food in the US compared to those in other countries where pleasure from food is more valued. He states, "there is a sense among many Americans that food is as much a poison as it is a nutrient, and that eating is almost as dangerous as not eating."[157] The most pleasure-oriented and the least health-oriented people of France—perhaps unsurprisingly—were found to spend more time eating while also eating less, to value the pleasures of the moment, and to enjoy more variety in food. Other cultures focus on the *experience* of eating, while we focus on the potential *consequences* of eating. Ironically, all that worry hasn't actually made us any healthier. In fact, the fear of food is more likely harming us, by depriving us of nutrients, adding to our allostatic load, and triggering backlash eating.[158]

There are many ways to bring pleasure into your meals, but the most important is simply pausing to ask yourself what sounds good before eating. How often do you ask yourself what you want to eat versus what you think you *should* eat? One exercise that I sometimes have my clients do is to complete a few days of a food, mood, and thought journal. When I started assigning this exercise, I was surprised to see just how many people struggled to answer the question, "What do you want to eat?" It was a realization of just how out of touch we are with pleasure. If you are struggling with this aspect of eating, revisit the chart "What Sounds Good?" in Chapter 2 for help tuning in to your food preferences. You might even consider taking a picture of it with your phone so you have access to it whenever you're at a restaurant.

In planning meals, don't forget the final member of The Gang. There are many ways to incorporate pleasure, such as using tasty sauces to flavor up foods, finishing off a meal with something sweet, not skimping on salt, adding cheese, experimenting with different spice and herb blends, and adding to your meal flavor boosters, like crumbled bacon, dried fruits, toasted nuts, olives, or sun-dried tomatoes.

Also, don't forget about a pleasurable food environment. While life sometimes demands that your meals be eaten on the run or in front of a computer, when you can, eat with others to add to the satisfaction factor. Even a meal of subpar food can be pleasurable when enjoyed over laughter and a good conversation.

Plate Planning for Satisfaction

What does it look like to include The Gang on your plate? For those who are more visual, these flexible plate planners may be helpful:

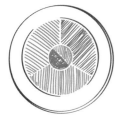

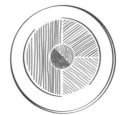

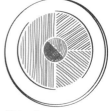

This plate is best for boosting protein and carbohydrate intake.

This plate is best for boosting produce intake while still getting adequate protein and carbohydrate.

This plate represents a meal that focuses more on carbohydrate while still incorporating adequate protein and produce.

 PROTEIN   CARBOHYDRATE   PRODUCE   FAT   PLEASURE

As you can see, there's no right or wrong. Intake of carbs, fat, protein, and produce will vary from meal to meal, depending on hunger levels, what sounds satisfying, planned activity level, and what food is available.

Keep in mind that while these plate planners can be helpful for some meals, they follow the more Eurocentric meal patterns that include a protein, a starch, and a vegetable. There are many perfectly balanced meals that don't look like any of these examples; mixed dishes, like curries, stir fries, or stews, may contain everything as well.

So, instead of trying to make your plate fit into a mold, I would encourage you to just aim to include The Gang, as that tends to create a most satisfying meal. This is just a recommendation and not a hard-and-fast rule. It's more helpful to use the concept of The Gang as a tool for getting curious about what feels good for you and anticipating future food needs.

Satisfying Snacks

To feel adequately fueled and energized throughout the day, most people need snacks. If you feel hungry between meals, you need a snack; it really is as simple as that. If you felt the urge to pee, you wouldn't question it, would you? So resist the urge to question your hunger. The alternative is to push off and suppress your hunger, which, as you've learned, would only make you ravenous at your next meal. That means you would be more likely to eat past what feels physically good or to make an impulsive food choice—or both.

There is no rule for how many snacks you need in a day. Let hunger be your guide. That said, if you know you're going to go longer than three to four hours between meals, it's smart to plan on having something available. Remember, your stomach empties after about this amount of time, and your blood sugar is likely to dip, so be prepared.

When you enjoy a snack, think beyond fruits and vegetables. Diet culture approaches snacking with the goal of filling up your stomach with the smallest number of calories, hence the recommendations for rice cakes, air-popped popcorn, and raw fruits and veggies. I don't know about you, but celery sticks or an apple will rarely address my immediate hunger, let alone tide me over for a couple hours. While it is certainly appropriate to include produce as *part* of a snack, unless you're about to eat a meal in a relatively short time, you'll want something more satisfying.

For a satisfying snack, it's helpful to pair a carbohydrate-containing food with something else that contains fat and/or protein. Generally speaking, if you include at least two food groups, you'll get this kind of balance. A carb paired with fat and/or protein helps stabilize blood sugar by providing your body with glucose, its essential fuel source, as well as other macronutrients. Again, this is a guideline, not a rule.

Meal and Snack Timing

I'm always amazed by just how confident some people are that *their* eating schedule is *the right* eating schedule. Rigid eating schedules ignore the fact that humans evolved to survive a food-insecure environment, where we couldn't ensure access to food every two hours or four hours or wait sixteen hours before eating to allow our bodies to fast. I don't think ancient humans were tracking the sun's position in the sky to see if it was time to eat yet. Any hard-and-fast rule about meal and snack timing simply isn't rooted in scientific evidence, and it doesn't account for human adaptability.

Even if one day science were able to agree on the "correct" schedule for eating, our busy modern life would make that schedule impossible to stick to. If you're anything like most

Satisfying Snacks

Looking for some snack inspirations? Here are fifteen easy ideas:

1. Top creamy full-fat yogurt with a handful of granola or bran cereal for crunch.

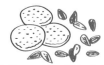

2. Toss a handful of cheese crackers with a handful of roasted almonds.

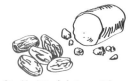

3. Stuff pitted dates with creamy goat cheese.

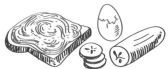

4. Make a savory version of ants on a log by filling celery sticks with hummus and topping them with chopped Kalamata olives.

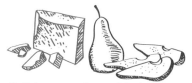

5. Top rice cakes with mashed avocado, crumbled goat cheese, and a little hot sauce or Sriracha.

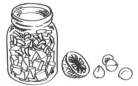

6. Pair a granola bar or protein bar with a piece of fresh fruit.

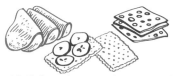

7. Spread a piece of toast with garlic hummus, cucumber slices, and diced hard-boiled egg; garnish with everything bagel seasoning.

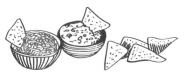

8. Enjoy pear slices with sharp cheddar cheese, or layer both on top of a slice of toasted pumpernickel bread spread with whole-grain mustard.

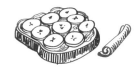

9. Toss pineapple or mango chunks with shredded coconut, lime juice, and chopped macadamia nuts.

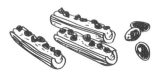

10. Enjoy wheat crackers topped with bread-and-butter pickle rounds, deli turkey or cheese, and a dollop of mustard.

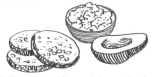

11. Have tortilla chips with guacamole and salsa; they make for an easy and satisfying combo. Look for individual guacamole containers for a packable snack.

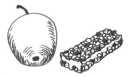

12. Spread your favorite nut butter on toast and top with banana slices and a sprinkle of cinnamon.

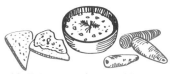

13. Enjoy pita chips and baby carrots with store-bought or homemade tzatziki.

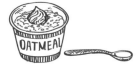

14. Warm up a cup of oatmeal and top it with a scoop of nut butter. I love to keep individual cups of oatmeal and peanut butter at my office for this snack.

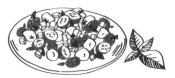

15. Make a caprese-inspired salad with mini mozzarella balls, cherry tomatoes, diced peaches, chopped basil, and a drizzle of balsamic vinegar.

of the people I work with, every day is different. This is especially true for shift workers, students, stay-at-home parents, or anyone with a nontraditional schedule. Sometimes the time you are able to stop and eat is dictated by when you can find a spare moment in the day.

In an ideal world for intuitive eating, you would be able to stop whenever you felt hungry, eat when you were in the mood to eat, and go about your day until you were hungry again. This sounds lovely, but it's not a reality for anyone I know. Living a real life with real responsibilities means you're not always able to stop what you're doing to eat, and when you do eat, you rarely have an array of choices. Sometimes it's food that has to fit your schedule instead of the other way around.

In addition to that, if you're healing from disordered eating or dealing with acute stress or the digestive issues that interfere with your body's natural hunger cues, you might not feel hunger, yet your body still needs fuel. If that describes you, you probably won't be eating adequately by looking to hunger as your sole prompt for eating.

This is where planning ahead and having a loose schedule for eating can be useful. While there's no one eating schedule that's right, your body still needs to be fed regularly in order to feel satisfied and energized and to give you the headspace to do the things you want to do. As a loose guideline, I'd encourage you to eat something every three to four hours, whether it is a meal or a snack. This aligns with our body's natural digestive rhythms, as toward the end of this period of time, your stomach will likely be empty. It's also around this time that blood sugar levels will start to dip, signaling the need for more food.

That said, sometimes you might need to eat more frequently than this, especially if you are very active or going through a growth period, like pregnancy or teenage years. Other times, it could be because the last thing you ate wasn't satisfying enough or because you're honoring practical hunger and not sure when you're going to get to eat again. And sometimes you might find yourself going longer than four hours, for example on a day you're less active or if your last meal was larger or consisted of particularly rich food.

Also, remember that if you're awake, your body needs food. If you work night shifts or tend to stay up late for one reason or another, you should be eating. Even if it means eating at hours that aren't considered "normal," I encourage you to still try not to go much longer than four hours without eating.

Meal Planning Versus Meal Preparedness

Part of honoring your hunger is making sure you have food available when hunger hits. This is where meal planning comes in handy. Without a plan, you're left making a decision about food when you're already feeling hungry. With glucose levels in the brain low, that decision is going to feel stressful and likely impulsive. Besides, if you have to go out to procure food and prepare it, you're likely going to be ravenous by the time you actually eat. It's challenging to incorporate gentle nutrition into making a food choice when you're already hungry, as your brain will focus on the immediate need of getting energy to it as quickly as possible. A hungry brain will fall back on old, habitual behaviors with food, whether it's a fast-food meal or zoning out with a box of cheese crackers in front of the TV. It's not that these choices are wrong—we've all had meals like this that are born out of hunger. It just probably doesn't feel great when that becomes your routine.

Meal planning continues the theme of things that could be useful, but have, unfortunately, been taken over by diet culture. When I search #mealprep on Instagram, I am bombarded with over 11 million images of meals perfectly portioned in matching plastic containers, almost half of which seem to be some combination of chicken or salmon, broccoli, and brown rice or sweet potatoes. When I search #mealplanning, I get almost a million images of organized, calorie-controlled plans and weekly spreadsheets with breakfast, lunch, dinner, and snacks in pretty fonts.

These rigid plans are the antithesis of intuitive eating, which involves listening to your body and considering what sounds good in the moment. I'm guessing what sounded good to you Sunday morning probably doesn't sound as tasty Thursday afternoon, especially when you've eaten the same meal for lunch four days in a row.

So, what's the middle ground? Not having a plan leads to impulsive food choices and getting overly hungry; having a plan that's too rigid doesn't leave space for flexibility and intuitive eating. This is where I'd like to introduce the concept I refer to as *meal preparedness*.

Meal preparedness is a more flexible way of meal planning. It means that you are prepared with meal and snack ideas as well as the foods and ingredients to be able to quickly feed yourself, but you also have enough flexibility and latitude to make a more specific decision about what you want to eat in the moment.

To practice meal preparedness, I encourage you to pick a day of the week to set aside a little time for planning. While it's helpful to have the same day each week to get into a routine, that may not always work for your schedule. The idea is that by looking ahead for the week, you're able to see any challenges and get a feel for how much time you might have for meal preparation. For example, what you might plan for a week that's packed with nighttime social engagements would look different from what you might plan for a week that has fewer evening commitments. It can also help you identify situations in which having a more structured plan in place might be helpful, for example, the evenings when your kids have after-school sports practice and you'd like to already have something prepared.

What meal preparedness looks like for you will vary based on your lifestyle, your cooking skills, and who else is eating in the household. But generally speaking, I encourage you to pick out two to four recipes or dishes for which you have the ingredients on hand. These can be new recipes you're excited to try or some old favorites that you could cook blindfolded. Keep in mind that a new recipe, no matter how easy it claims to be, will always take more time, as you'll be looking back at the recipe while cooking.

Having a few planned meals as well as some fallback options both provides the security of having foods available at home and leaves space for making intuitive decisions about food depending on what you're in the mood for.

Stocking Your Kitchen for Gentle Nutrition

Part of meal preparedness is being stocked with kitchen staples—ingredients that are shelf stable or will last more than a week or two in your pantry or fridge. This lets you throw together easy meals and be flexible with food without making a million trips to the grocery store. The following list gives you some ideas to get started.

PANTRY

PASTA
Pasta is great for throwing together an easy and satisfying meal. Just add a store-bought sauce, sautéed or frozen vegetables, and a pantry protein, like canned tuna, a crumbled veggie burger, or canned beans.

GRAINS
I like to have different grains on hand. Some grains, like brown rice or farro take a long time to cook, so I recommend having some quick-cooking whole grains, like quinoa or white rice, for weeknight meals.

BOXED PASTA, RICE, OR GRAIN MIXES
Whether it's boxed mac and cheese or a seasoned rice or quinoa mix, these convenient foods make for a simple and tasty side dish or something to add to the rest of The Gang to create a satisfying meal.

OATS
Oats are more versatile than you imagine. Having a bag of rolled oats around is great for making a quick breakfast of oatmeal or overnight oats, but you can also add them to smoothies for fiber and filling carbs, put them in muffins or cookies, or blend them with nut butter and honey to make energy balls.

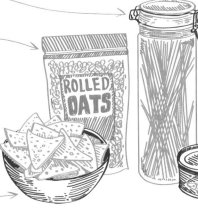 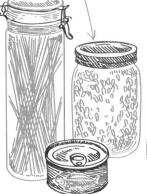 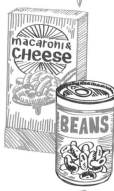

TORTILLA CHIPS
Between eating them as snacks and incorporating them into an entrée, I go through a big bag of tortilla chips each week. You can also add cheese, beans, and sautéed veggies to them to make easy nachos.

CANNED TUNA, SALMON, OR SARDINES
To quickly add protein to a meal, it's hard to beat canned fish. Packed with omega-3 fats, calcium, and vitamin D, canned fish is a nutrient-rich choice. Mix the fish with olive oil, lemon juice, and herbs, and enjoy it with crackers as a snack.

CANNED BEANS
You can't beat the convenience of canned beans. They are an easy and inexpensive way to round out simple meals. I almost always have canned chickpeas, black beans, and cannellini beans on hand, along with a can of refried beans for a simple side dish or for snacking on with tortilla chips.

CANNED ENTRÉES

Don't be afraid of canned goods. Remember, processed foods can make healthy eating more convenient. I like to have canned Indian food, like dal or palak paneer; chili; and a soup or two available. You can enjoy these canned entrées on their own or round them out to a more satisfying meal by bringing in shelf-stable carbs, like canned chili stuffed into a baked sweet potato or canned palak paneer served over rice.

ONIONS AND GARLIC

Onions and garlic are versatile flavor powerhouses. Store them in a cool, dark place to prevent them from molding.

COCONUT MILK:

Canned coconut milk is essential for making the creamiest oatmeal. You can also use it to make curry sauce, to make smoothies more satiating, or to add creaminess to sauces and soups.

OILS

I use olive oil and either canola or avocado oil as everyday cooking oils, but it's also nice to have other oils on hand to add flavor, like peanut or sesame oil for stir-fries, walnut oil for salad dressing, or coconut oil for baking.

SPICES AND DRIED HERBS

Spices and dried herbs are indispensable in my kitchen. If you don't feel comfortable combining spices on your own, or if you don't have much storage, go for the various spice blends.

DRIED FRUITS

Keep an assortment of dried fruits as a flavor booster for salads, a topping for oatmeal or roasted vegetables, or to add to savory rice dishes. Dried fruits are also a great pantry staple snack, paired with a handful of nuts.

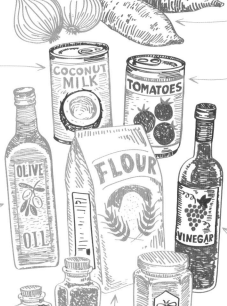

FLOURS

All-purpose flour is essential (or gluten-free flour, if needed), as is whole wheat flour if you're baking with whole grains. You can also get creative baking with different whole-grain or alternative flours, like almond flour, spelt flour, cornmeal, or oat flour.

NUTS AND NUT BUTTER

What's great about nuts is that for the most part, they are pretty interchangeable, which makes them a versatile flavor booster for both sweet and savory dishes. While I have them listed as a pantry ingredient, I keep mine in the freezer, which keeps the oils from going rancid.

POTATOES

I like to have sweet potatoes and a couple of varieties of waxy potatoes to use in a breakfast hash, to add to soups or stews, or to roast up with salt, pepper, and rosemary for a classic, simple side.

CANNED TOMATOES AND TOMATO SAUCE

I use canned tomatoes at least once a week to make pastas, soups, or curries. Jarred tomato sauce is also a tasty ingredient for braising chicken, cod or other mild white fish, or vegetables, like green beans or zucchini.

VINEGARS

Having a bottle each of red or white wine vinegar, apple cider vinegar, balsamic, and rice vinegar in the pantry will get you through most recipes.

SWEETENERS

I skip the artificial sweeteners and go for the real stuff; it tastes much better. Table sugar, brown sugar, honey, and maple syrup should cover the basics.

FREEZER

FROZEN MEALS
Whether it's pizzas, burritos, or skillet meals, some days you need a meal that requires nothing more than a few minutes in the microwave or quick toast in the oven. I always try to have two or three options on hand for the days I'm running out the door.

FROZEN VEGETABLES
Frozen vegetables are just as nutritious as fresh and, since vegetables are frozen at peak ripeness, they often contain more nutrients in comparison to fresh produce, which loses nutrients over time during transit from the farm to the grocery store, and then to your fridge where it continues to sit.[159] Having a few frozen vegetables on hand keeps you from needing to go to the grocery store all the time.

FROZEN FRENCH FRIES OR TATER TOTS
Serving french fries or tater tots as your carbohydrate source as part of a regular dinner helps to normalize fried foods. Also, it might sound odd, but I love to add sweet potato fries to salads.

FROZEN FRUITS
For a light and fresh breakfast or snack, frozen fruits are essential for smoothies.

FROZEN BREAD
Keep some bread in the freezer. It's always nice to have a backup loaf in case you run out.

VEGGIE BURGERS
I love to have veggie burgers on hand to crumble into salads, pasta dishes, and grain bowls to boost protein. Try different brands to see if there's one you prefer.

BACON
Bacon is a great way to add flavor to vegetables, soups, and salads. I separate bacon into individual slices, roll them up like fruit roll-ups, and freeze them. This way I can use a slice or two as needed.

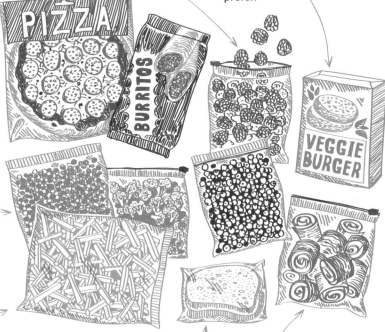

REFRIGERATOR

EGGS
When in doubt, throw an egg on it. Topping a bowl of pasta or toast and sautéed veggies or even canned soup with an egg—fried, soft-boiled, or poached—is my favorite way to round out a quick meal.

MILK
Whether it's for making smoothies or oatmeal, or for enjoying with cookies, it's smart to have milk on hand. Go with what you enjoy—dairy, almond, oat, soy, etc.

YOGURT
While I love flavored yogurt for its convenience, I usually keep a tub of full-fat plain yogurt on hand for cooking or to serve sweetened with jam, honey, or fruits as a snack.

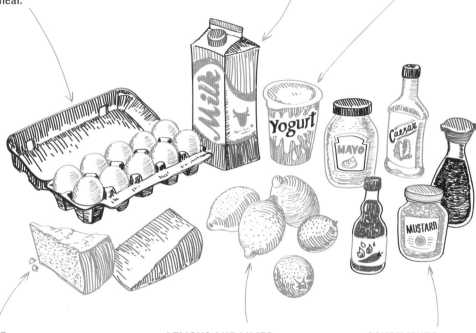

CHEESE
While soft cheeses spoil more quickly, two of the more versatile cheeses, cheddar and Parmesan, last longer—about a month for a block of cheddar and seven to nine months for Parmesan.

LEMONS AND LIMES
Lemons and limes add the essential element of acid to meals. If my lemons or limes are starting to get a little hard and dried out, I zest and juice them and freeze each in separate containers.

CONDIMENTS
I'm a bit of a condiment hoarder. When I purchased a new refrigerator, storage space in the doors was the most important thing to me. If forced to choose, salad dressing, soy sauce, hot sauce, mustard, and mayo should cover the very basics. To dress up your go-to recipes and keep them interesting, I'd encourage you to pick up a new sauce or condiment when you do your regular grocery shopping.

Cooking for Satisfaction

You may have read these past few sections and thought, "That's great and all, but I am not a cook." If so, that's okay. Intuitive eating and gentle nutrition do not require gourmet cooking skills—or *any* cooking skills. There are so many tasty, nutritious, and satisfying meals that are just a few minutes in the microwave, a phone call, or a trip to a deli away.

Part of why you dislike or avoid cooking may be diet culture. If you've only cooked based on what you think you should be eating, cooking probably feels like a chore to you. Similarly, trying to prepare meals on nights you really don't have the time but are too afraid to eat a microwave meal or takeout will take the joy out of cooking as well. Just as you can't make yourself enjoy movement by forcing yourself to exercise, you can't make yourself enjoy cooking by forcing yourself to cook.

That said, I do think cooking can be a powerful tool for making peace with food and for nourishing your body. As someone who has always enjoyed cooking, I admit I may be biased. However, the joy I've witnessed in many of my clients when they prepare a satisfying meal that focuses on pleasure and not the expectations of diet culture tells me that I might be on to something.

To me, cooking for satisfaction is a powerful, health-enhancing tool. It gives me a chance to relax at the end of a busy workday and connect with my husband as we cook together. Preparing dishes associated with happy times or vacations past is a way of fondly reminiscing. Getting curious about and trying new-to-me dishes from other cultures is a way to learn about and celebrate those cultures. Providing my body with nourishing home-cooked food is a way of treating my body with respect. At the very least, cooking is a way to simply enjoy a yummy meal.

So, in the next part, I introduce fifty recipes that focus on satisfaction and incorporate nutrition in a gentle way. Feeding yourself is an act of self-care, and putting some time into preparing something nourishing and tasty is one way to treat your body with kindness and hopefully bring joy into your life. Getting your hands dirty in the kitchen helps you normalize foods and build a healthier relationship with them. Just as building an appreciation for what your body can do helps you feel more peaceful with it, building an appreciation for what different foods can do helps you feel more peaceful with them. I hope that by viewing meal planning and cooking through a more flexible lens, you'll come to see these health-promoting practices as being more accessible to you.

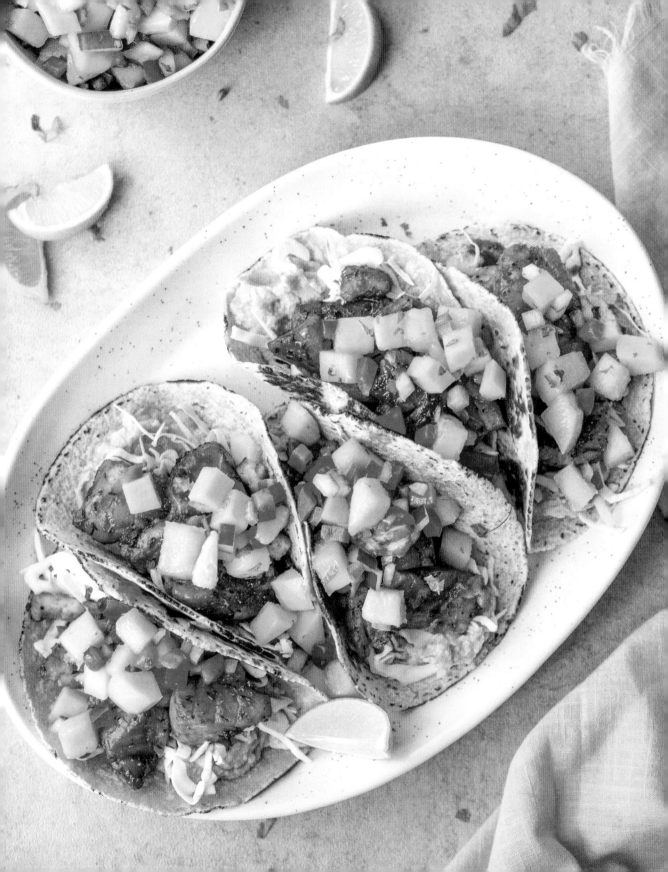

Part 2
THE
RECIPES

When I started a food blog in 2013, if you'd asked me what my approach to cooking was, I would have said I believed that all foods fit and that healthy food could and should taste good. However, when I look back at my early recipes, I don't see that philosophy. Most of what I see are attempts to make dishes "healthier" through eliminating or reducing the ingredients that I thought were "unhealthy" or through making "clean eating" swaps. Nutrition and "health" came first; taste came second.

Today, when I develop recipes, my focus is first and foremost on pleasure and what I want to eat. Once that's in place, I think about adding in nutrition in a way that is gentle and enhances taste as opposed to sacrificing it. I approach fruits, vegetables, whole grains, and other nutrient-packed ingredients as a way of adding flavors and textures rather than as filler foods or swaps.

The recipes in this book follow this newer approach. To develop them, I started with a list of the foods I love and the recipes I make again and again at home. I also thought about convenience and worked to come up with recipes that accommodate easy meal prep and feeding yourself on busy nights. I hope cooking these recipes will help strengthen your understanding of gentle nutrition and what it looks like to nourish both your mind and your body.

I've suggested quantities of ingredients for ease of shopping and typical serving sizes to help with planning, but please remember that you are free to honor your appetite. Use more or less of an ingredient as you desire, and eat as much of a dish as you like. These recipes and serving sizes are just a guide. It's how hungry you are when you make it, your biological food needs, as well as how you are serving a dish (with or without sides) that determine how many servings a recipe really makes. There is no right or wrong amount to eat.

To make the recipes accessible to the widest range of people, I occasionally include suggestions for making a recipe gluten-free, vegetarian, vegan, or allergy-friendly, as long as it doesn't compromise the integrity of the dish. I understand that many people have dietary restrictions for medical or ethical reasons. If that's you, I want to open up as many of these recipes as possible for you! If not, please know that these recommendations are not to make a recipe "healthier" or compatible with any weight loss diet.

Lastly, feel free to get creative with these recipes. I view cooking as an art, not a science. It's a place to experiment and play, not a list of rules to follow by the book. When appropriate, I've offered suggestions to switch things up. Once you feel comfortable with a cooking technique, a world of options opens up! Remember, with food, there's no right or wrong. Follow the late, great Julia Child's advice: "Learn how to cook—try new recipes, learn from your mistakes, be fearless, and above all have fun!"

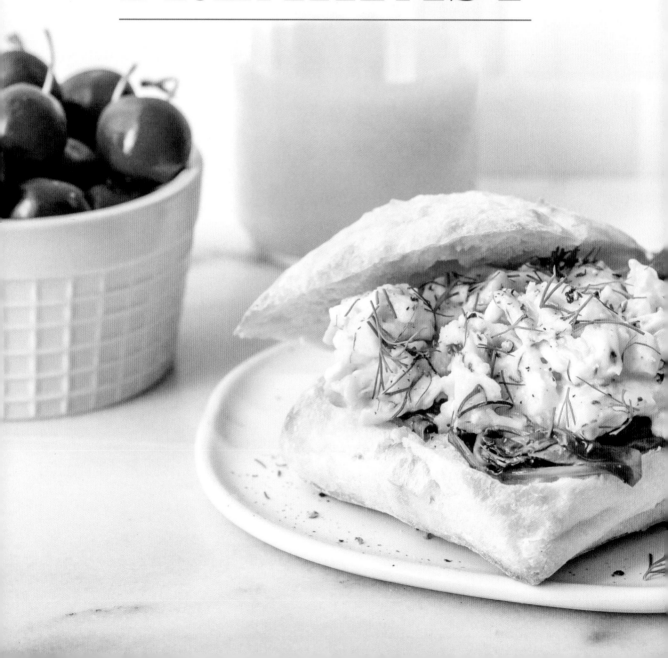

Chapter 7
BREAKFAST

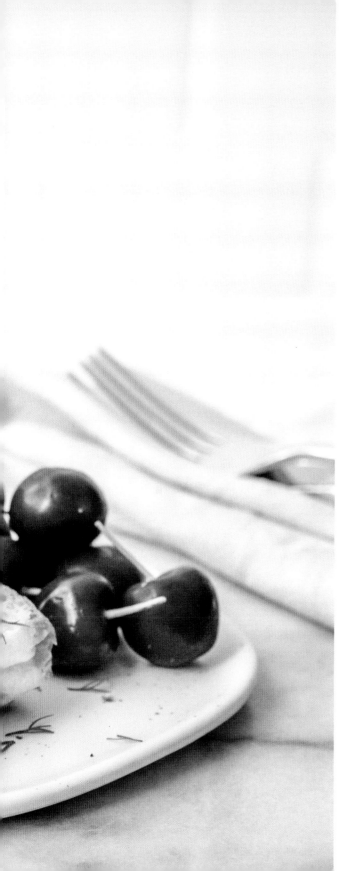

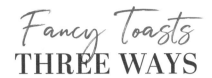

Fancy Toasts
THREE WAYS

MAKES 2 slices PREP TIME: 5 minutes COOK TIME: 5 minutes

When you're running out the door in the morning, it's hard to beat the simplicity of toast. When it comes to providing that fullness factor, however, toast is simply not going to power you through the morning. I can't tell you how many of my clients have reported binge eating at night or low energy during the day only to tell me that they typically eat just a slice or two of toast for breakfast. Remember the rest of The Gang? Don't leave your toast hanging out alone!

Thankfully, avocado toast has ignited the fancy toast trend—something I can definitely get behind. Adding fats and protein to a crusty piece of toasted bread makes it a satisfying breakfast that you can prep in minutes. If you like, pair any of these toasts with fresh fruit, yogurt, or another side to round out your meal.

Crunchy PBJ Toast

Crunchy granola and seeds give basic peanut butter toast an upgrade. Feel free to play around with different flavor combinations, like chocolate granola and cherry jam or vanilla granola with blueberry jam. Don't be afraid of nut butter. It is more energy-dense, but it also is packed with nutrition and provides major satisfaction factor. The amount I've listed here is just a suggestion; whether you use peanut butter for the classic PBJ flavor or other nut butters, like almond or cashew, feel free to layer it on the toast nice and thick and to have a slice or two for a snack.

2 slices nutty, seedy whole-grain bread

2 tablespoons peanut butter

1 tablespoon jam

2 to 3 tablespoons granola

1 teaspoon chia or flax seeds (optional)

1. Toast the bread as desired.

2. Spread the toast with the peanut butter, followed by the jam (feel free to use more or less peanut butter or jam depending on preference and the size of your bread). Sprinkle with the granola and chia or flax seeds, if using, and serve.

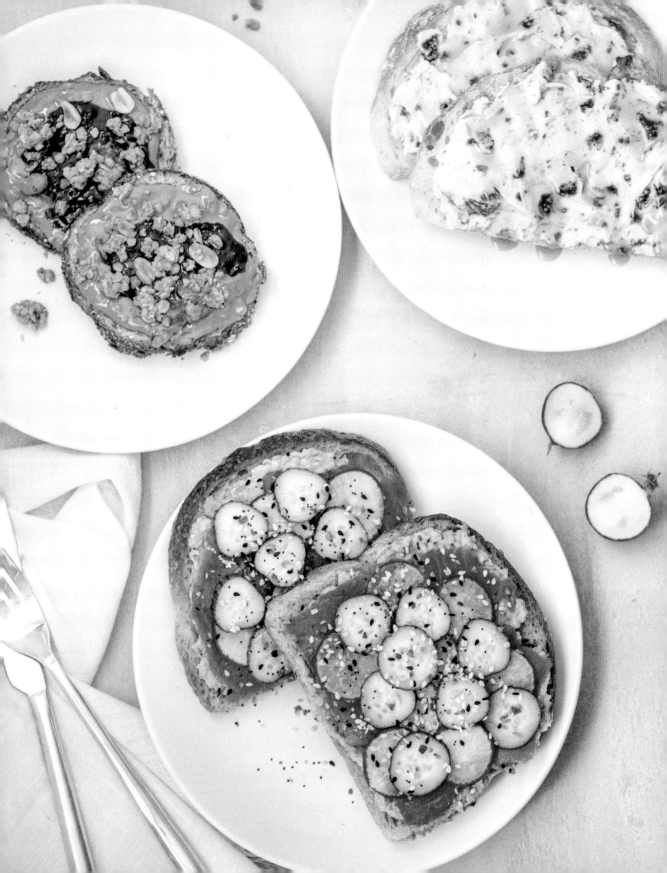

Fruit and Cream Cheese Toast

This fancy toast was inspired by the classic combination of dried fruits and creamy goat cheeses served on cheese boards. I often prep a larger batch of the fruit and cheese spread to shorten breakfast prep or to enjoy as a snack with crackers. Dried figs and dates are my favorite fruits to use in this spread, but I've also made it with dried cherries, apricots, and cranberries. For best results, use rustic, crusty bread, such as boule.

2 slices crusty bread

2 tablespoons cream cheese

2 tablespoons goat cheese

1 tablespoon chopped dried dates

1 tablespoon chopped dried figs

Honey, for drizzling

1. Toast the bread as desired.

2. In a small bowl, mix together the cream cheese, goat cheese, dates, and figs until combined. Spread over the toast, drizzle with honey, and serve.

Smoked Salmon Avocado Toast

Smoked salmon and avocado are two of my all-time favorite foods, which makes this toast one of my all-time favorite breakfasts! Smoked salmon adds a boost of omega-3 fats, while radish and cucumber add crunch.

2 slices sourdough bread

½ to 1 avocado, halved, pitted, and peeled

A few slices smoked salmon

A few thin slices cucumber

A few thin slices radish

Everything bagel seasoning, for sprinkling

1. Toast the bread as desired.

2. Top each slice with ¼ to ½ avocado and mash it into the toast with the back of a fork. Top with a couple slices of smoked salmon and a few slices of cucumber and radish. Sprinkle lightly with everything bagel seasoning and serve.

Gingery Blueberry
BANANA SMOOTHIE

MAKES 1 smoothie   PREP TIME: 5 minutes

Smoothies are a great option when you want to start your day with something light and fresh—or if you don't have much of an appetite in the morning. But let's not think of smoothies as a way to fill up your stomach with as few calories as possible. Being liquid, smoothies are inherently less filling, as they are digested faster than foods consumed in solid form. For this reason, you want to be mindful about including the whole gang. This refreshing breakfast gets a little carbohydrate and extra fiber from rolled oats, which blend right into the smoothie, adding a nice creamy texture. It also gets a dose of fat and protein from almond butter. You could pair this smoothie with buttered toast, oatmeal, or one of the egg muffins on pages 142 to 145 for an even more satisfying breakfast.

1 cup frozen blueberries

½ large banana, frozen, cut into chunks

1 (1-inch) piece ginger, peeled and grated

3 tablespoons rolled oats

1½ tablespoons almond butter

1 cup whole or 2% milk

Honey (optional, to sweeten)

Place all the ingredients in a blender and blend until completely smooth. Serve immediately.

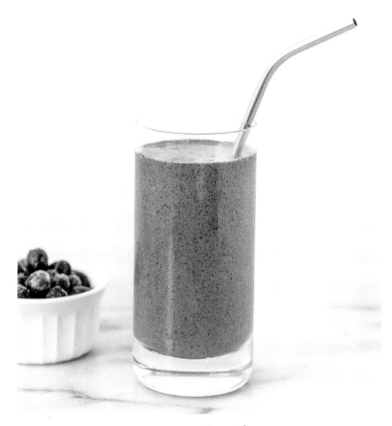

Perfect Scrambled EGGS IN A BASKET

MAKES 1 serving   PREP TIME: 5 minutes   COOK TIME: 10 minutes

There's nothing like soft and creamy scrambled eggs fresh out of the skillet (except maybe for a perfectly poached egg, but that's a technique I have yet to master!). The key is to cook your eggs low and slow, which makes them fluffy and moist with a silky texture. Cooking eggs over higher heat toughens the proteins, making the eggs taste rubbery and dry. I prefer my scrambled eggs a little wet, but feel free to cook yours until completely set; just be sure to stop before they get hard and dry.

Another key to this recipe is butter. I love the flavor of olive oil, but when it comes to scrambled eggs, butter is better. Besides, the scent of nutty melted butter filling your kitchen in the morning is most heavenly!

I like to break out this recipe on a weekend or, more often, make it as an easy breakfast-for-dinner meal. Once you get the hang of scrambling the eggs, this dish is likely to become a weeknight staple paired with sautéed vegetables. Spread the top of the roll with butter and jam for a sweet finish.

1 ciabatta roll

2 teaspoons unsalted butter, divided

1 clove garlic, minced

2 handfuls fresh baby spinach (about 2 ounces)

Salt and black pepper

2 large eggs, beaten until slightly frothy

1 tablespoon chopped herbs, like dill, parsley, or chives, plus extra for garnish

Crumbled goat cheese or feta cheese

1. Preheat the oven to 350°F.

2. Cut the ciabatta roll in half. To make a well for the spinach and eggs, pull out a little bit of the bread from the center of the bottom half. (Freeze or refrigerate the pulled-out bread for making breadcrumbs later.) Toast both halves of the roll in the oven until golden and crispy, 6 to 8 minutes.

3. Meanwhile, melt 1 teaspoon of the butter in a small nonstick skillet over medium heat. Add the garlic and cook until fragrant, about 30 seconds. Stir in the spinach along with a pinch of salt and pepper and cook until wilted, about 2 minutes. When the ciabatta halves are done, fill the well with the sautéed spinach.

4. Reduce the heat to low, wipe the skillet clean, and add the remaining 1 teaspoon of butter to the skillet. Season the beaten eggs with a pinch of salt and pepper. Stir in the herbs. When the butter has melted, pour the egg mixture into the center of the skillet and swirl it around to coat. When the eggs look slightly thickened and just barely set at the edges, use a silicone spatula to push the edges toward the center to let the uncooked eggs flood the skillet. Continue this process until the eggs are soft and creamy with large curds but still a little wet.

5. Stir in the cheese and cook until it melts, about 15 seconds. If the eggs still look a little wet, don't worry; there will be some carryover cooking in the skillet, off the heat.

6. Scoop the eggs on top of the spinach and sprinkle with a bit of salt and pepper. Garnish with more fresh herbs, if desired. Serve immediately.

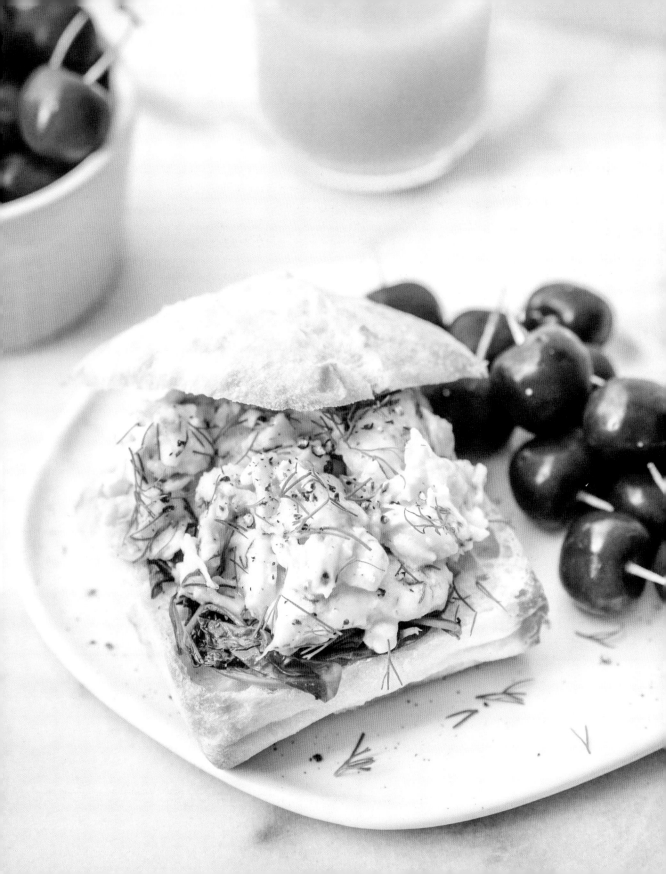

Whole-Grain Cinnamon-Apple
STREUSEL MUFFINS

———— MAKES 12 muffins PREP TIME: 15 minutes COOK TIME: 30 minutes ————

Baking is generally not my forte, but I must say these muffins are easily the finest to come out of my kitchen. Their texture is dense and hearty yet moist, with a bit of crunch from the granola. And the aroma of cinnamon and apple wafting from the oven is just heavenly.

Muffins provide a great platform for the nutty flavor of whole grains to shine, and this makes them a great way to introduce these nutrient-rich ingredients. However, the fiber in whole grains, though filling, tends to make baked goods dry and coarse. So, while many "health food" or "clean eating" recipes call for all whole-grain flour, I usually use half white flour and half whole-grain flour—as I do here—to keep baked goods tender. For this recipe, I also let the batter rest for ten to twenty minutes before baking to get the whole-wheat flour hydrated and, therefore, softened.

I enjoy these muffins alongside creamy Greek yogurt topped with fresh fruit for breakfast. They're also great as a snack, especially spread with a bit of nut butter. The muffins are also freezer-friendly; just warm a frozen muffin for about thirty seconds in the microwave. This recipe can be made with gluten-free baking flour without any other modifications.

½ cup (1 stick) unsalted butter, melted

½ cup pure maple syrup

2 teaspoons vanilla extract

½ cup buttermilk or kefir

½ cup plain whole-milk or 2% Greek yogurt

2 large eggs

1 cup all-purpose flour

1 cup whole-wheat flour

2½ teaspoons baking powder

½ teaspoon baking soda

½ teaspoon ground cinnamon

½ teaspoon salt

1 large apple (any type), cored and diced

2 cups granola, divided

1. Preheat the oven to 350°F. Grease a standard-size 12-cup muffin tin or line with paper liners.

2. In a large mixing bowl, whisk together the butter, maple syrup, and vanilla extract until combined. Whisk in the buttermilk, yogurt, and eggs until homogenous. In a medium bowl, whisk together the flours, baking powder, baking soda, cinnamon, and salt. Add the dry ingredients into the wet ingredients; stir with a spoon or a rubber spatula until just combined. Fold in the diced apple and 1 cup of the granola.

3. Divide the batter evenly among the wells of the muffin tin. Sprinkle the remaining 1 cup of granola evenly over the batter and press it down lightly. Bake until a toothpick inserted into the middle of a muffin comes out clean, 25 to 30 minutes. Let cool in the pan for 10 minutes. Unmold and transfer to a rack to cool completely. Store the muffins in a covered container at room temperature for up to 2 days or for up to a week in the fridge.

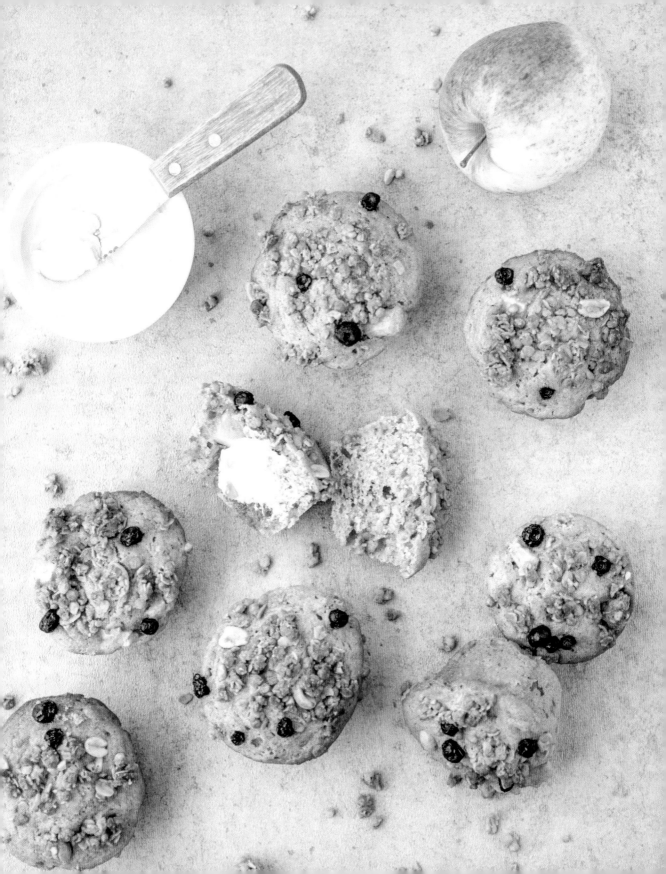

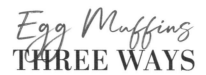

Egg Muffins
THREE WAYS

MAKES 12 muffins   PREP TIME: 10 minutes   COOK TIME: 30 minutes

I rarely get my act together enough on a Sunday to do meal prep, but when I do, egg muffins are a must. As a perpetual snooze button–hitter, I eat most of my breakfasts while multitasking—putting on my makeup or working at my computer. So it's great to have something tasty and satisfying that I can grab and go.

These egg muffins couldn't be easier to make. You start with a basic batter that invites you to experiment with any fillings you like. (I've included three of my favorite combinations here.) The muffins will last up to five days in the refrigerator, or you can freeze the cooled muffins for three to four months in a large zip-top bag or plastic or glass container labeled with the date. To serve, pull out one or two at a time and heat them up for thirty to sixty seconds in the microwave.

I love to use these egg muffins to make an easy breakfast sandwich with an English muffin, split and toasted. They're also great paired with fresh fruit and toast or hash browns.

Shiitake and Thyme

1 tablespoon extra-virgin olive oil

½ large yellow onion, finely diced

Pinch of salt

1 clove garlic, minced

8 ounces fresh shiitake mushrooms, trimmed and sliced

½ teaspoon chopped thyme leaves

1 cup crumbled goat cheese

EGG MUFFIN BATTER:

8 large eggs

¼ cup whole or 2% milk

¼ teaspoon salt

¼ teaspoon cracked black pepper

1. Preheat the oven to 375°F. Grease a standard-size 12-cup muffin tin.

2. Heat the olive oil in a large skillet over medium-high heat. Add the onion and salt and cook, stirring occasionally, until the onion is translucent, about 3 minutes. Stir in the garlic, mushrooms, and thyme and cook until the mushrooms are tender and golden, about 5 minutes.

3. Meanwhile, prepare the egg muffin batter by whisking together the eggs, milk, salt, and pepper.

4. Divide the mushroom mixture evenly among the wells of the muffin tin. Divide the egg muffin batter evenly among the wells. Sprinkle the goat cheese over the top. Bake until the tops are golden brown and the eggs feel firm when pressed, about 20 minutes.

Everything Bagel Smoked Salmon

1 tablespoon extra-virgin olive oil

1 cup halved cherry tomatoes

4 ounces smoked salmon, chopped

3 scallions, thinly sliced

2 tablespoons chopped dill

1 tablespoon small capers in brine, drained

¼ cup (2 ounces) cream cheese, divided

Everything bagel seasoning

1. Preheat the oven to 375°F. Grease a standard-size 12-cup muffin tin.

2. Heat the olive oil in a large skillet over medium-high heat. Add the tomatoes and cook until tender, 4 to 5 minutes. Add the smoked salmon, scallions, and dill and cook until cooked through, 1 to 2 minutes. Turn off the heat and stir in the capers.

3. Meanwhile, prepare the egg muffin batter as directed, opposite.

4. Divide the smoked salmon mixture among the wells of the muffin tin. Divide the egg muffin batter evenly among the wells. Top each with 1 teaspoon of the cream cheese and sprinkle with a bit of everything bagel seasoning. Bake until the tops are golden and the eggs feel firm when pressed, about 20 minutes.

Apple, Ham, and Cheddar

1 tablespoon extra-virgin olive oil

½ large sweet onion, finely diced

1 clove garlic, minced

Pinch of salt

1 large Gala or Fuji apple, cored and diced

7 ounces ham, diced

¾ cup shredded sharp cheddar cheese, divided

1. Preheat the oven to 375°F. Grease a standard-size 12-cup muffin tin.

2. Heat the olive oil in a large skillet over medium-high heat. Add the onion, garlic, and salt and cook, stirring occasionally, until the onion is translucent, 3 to 4 minutes. Stir in the apple and ham; cook, stirring occasionally, until the apple is tender, about 5 minutes. Set aside.

3. Meanwhile, prepare the egg muffin batter as directed, opposite.

4. Divide the apple and ham mixture evenly among the wells of the muffin tin. Divide the egg muffin batter evenly among the wells. Top each with 1 tablespoon of the shredded cheddar. Bake until the tops are golden and the eggs feel firm when pressed, about 20 minutes.

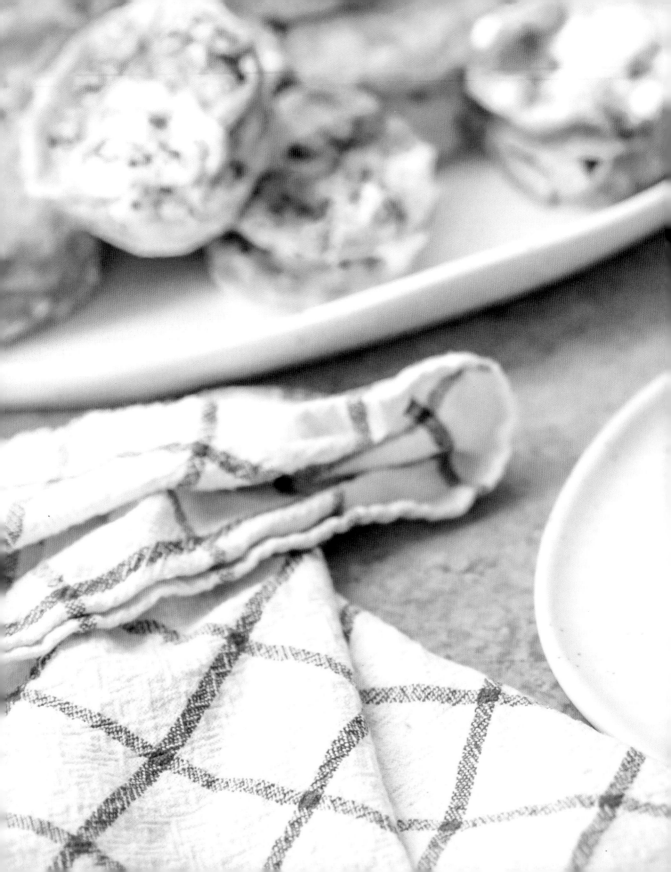

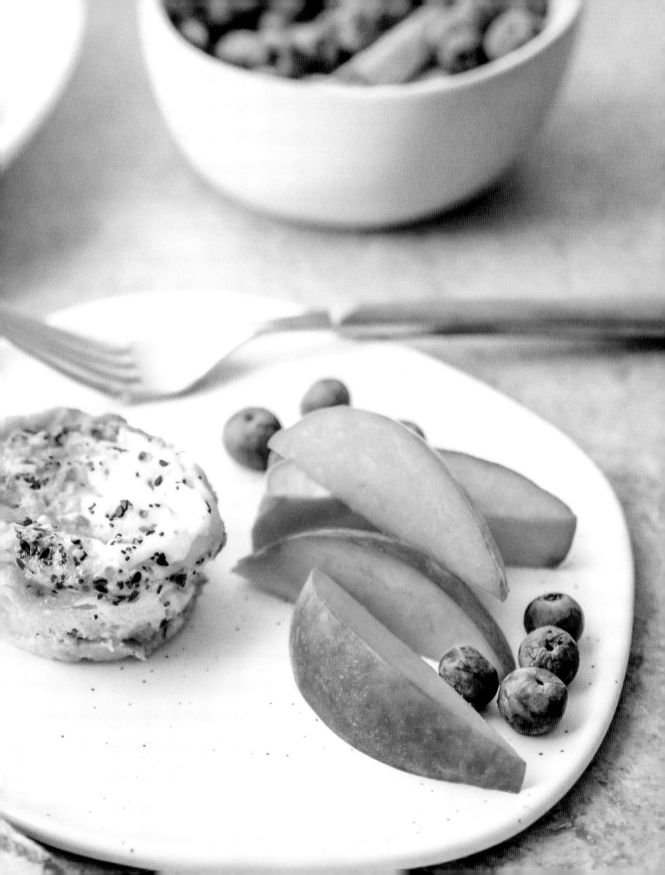

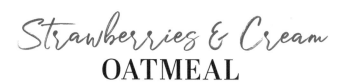

Strawberries & Cream
OATMEAL

MAKES 2 to 3 servings PREP TIME: 10 minutes COOK TIME: 15 minutes

I used to think I hated oatmeal. I thought it was bland and boring—the thing you forced yourself to eat when you were trying to be "good." Eventually, I learned that I just didn't know how to cook oatmeal, and that it could actually be creamy and flavorful with a slightly toothsome texture.

This recipe incorporates a few of my favorite oatmeal tricks. First, it calls for toasting the oats in coconut oil or butter. This improves the texture of the oats and brings out their natural flavor. Next, it calls for cooking the oats in a combination of coconut milk and water. While the more common method of cooking oats in milk adds flavor, it also makes them gluey and sticky from the milk proteins. Using coconut milk not only adds flavor and satisfying fats to the oats, but also helps their texture. Lastly, I flavor the oats by putting sugar, salt, and vanilla right into the cooking liquid instead of on top of the finished oatmeal. This way, the flavor seeps into the oats instead of hanging out on the surface.

I kick this oatmeal up even more by topping it with macerated strawberries. These are made by letting fresh strawberries sit in a bit of sugar, a process that both softens the strawberries and draws the juice out of them. This delicious juice will meld into the creamy oatmeal, sweetening it even further.

If you have leftover oatmeal, store it in the fridge. The oatmeal will thicken upon storage, so thin it out with a couple tablespoons of water when you reheat it in the microwave or on the stovetop.

MACERATED STRAWBERRIES:

1 cup fresh strawberries, hulled and quartered

1 tablespoon granulated sugar

OATMEAL:

1 teaspoon coconut oil or unsalted butter

1 cup rolled oats

1 cup canned full-fat or light coconut milk

1 cup water

1 tablespoon granulated sugar

1½ teaspoons vanilla extract

Large pinch of salt

FOR SERVING:

Chopped toasted pistachios

Plain or vanilla whole-milk or 2% Greek yogurt

1. Macerate the strawberries: Toss the berries with the sugar and set aside to soften and release the juice, about 10 minutes.

2. Meanwhile, heat the coconut oil in a medium saucepan over medium heat. Add the oats and cook, stirring occasionally, until they smell toasty and look slightly golden, about 5 minutes. Add the coconut milk, water, sugar, vanilla extract, and salt. Simmer, stirring occasionally, until creamy, 5 to 10 minutes.

3. Transfer to a bowl. Top the oatmeal with the macerated strawberries, pistachios, and yogurt.

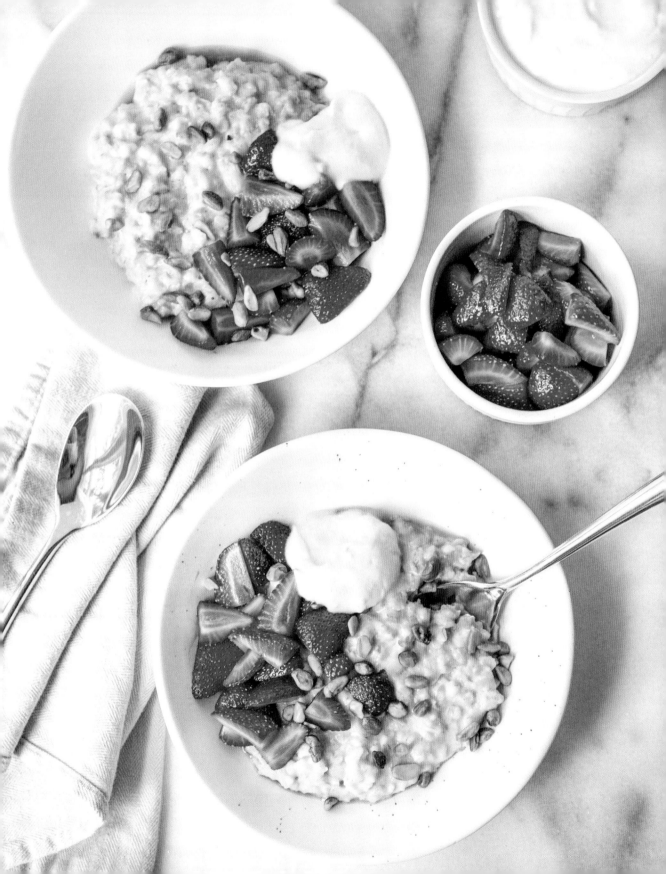

MIGAS

MAKES 2 servings   PREP TIME: 15 minutes   COOK TIME: 5 minutes

Migas is a traditional Mexican dish designed to turn leftover corn tortillas into a hearty breakfast. It's made by frying strips of tortillas until crispy, then adding eggs to make a scrambled mix.

In our house, we make migas Tex-Mex style—with onions, tomatoes, and jalapeño—for breakfast at least once a week and sometimes almost every day! As a time-saver, this recipe uses tortilla chips, which I always have on hand for snacking. Served over canned refried black beans—another kitchen staple— with tons of garnishes, it's one of those hearty and satisfying yet quick and budget-friendly meals I never tire of. When I want to save even more time (or when I don't feel like chopping vegetables), I often go for a simplified version with just eggs and tortilla chips, topped with hot sauce.

4 large eggs

1 tablespoon whole or 2% milk

Salt and black pepper

1 tablespoon extra-virgin olive oil

¼ cup diced onions

¼ cup diced tomatoes

½ jalapeño pepper, deseeded and finely diced

1 clove garlic, minced

2 large handfuls tortilla chips, lightly crushed

Canned refried black beans, warmed

FOR SERVING (OPTIONAL):

Sliced avocado

Chopped cilantro

Chopped scallions

Hot sauce or salsa

Crumbled feta cheese or queso fresco

1. In a medium bowl, whisk together the eggs and milk until frothy. Season with a pinch of salt and pepper and set aside.

2. Heat the olive oil in a medium skillet over medium heat. Add the onions, tomatoes, jalapeño, and garlic along with a pinch of salt. Cook until the onions are translucent, 3 to 4 minutes.

3. Pour the beaten eggs into the skillet and cook, pushing the edges toward the center, until the eggs are soft-scrambled but still wet. Stir in the tortilla chips and cook for another 30 seconds.

4. Serve the migas over the refried black beans. Serve with avocado, cilantro, scallions, hot sauce, and/or cheese, if desired.

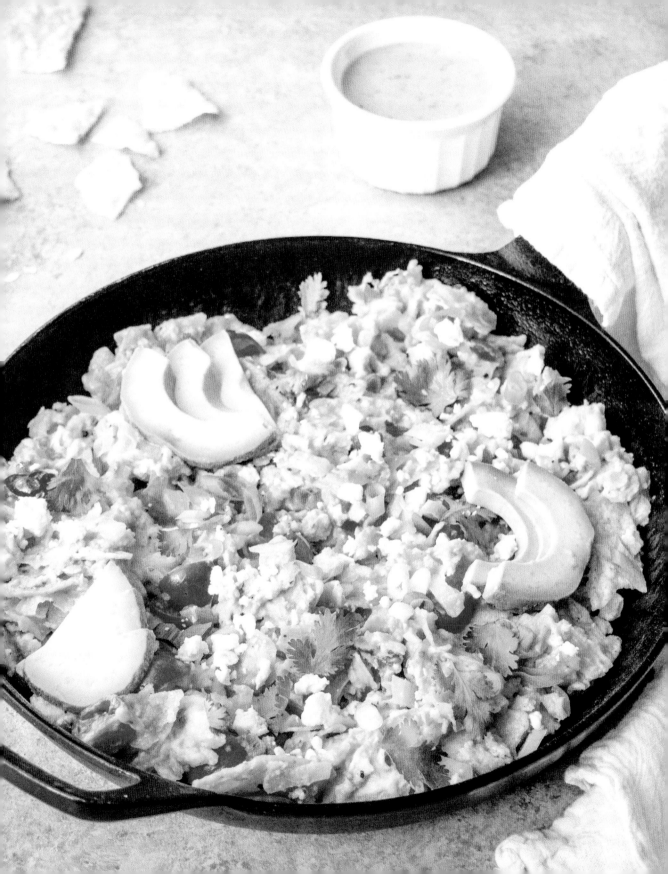

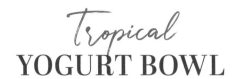

Tropical YOGURT BOWL

—— **MAKES** 1 serving   **PREP TIME:** 5 minutes ——

I can't tell you how many of my clients have told me they start their day with a cup of yogurt topped with a sprinkle of granola. That's great for a snack, but not so great for a meal. No wonder they're ravenous and miserable before lunchtime rolls around.

Yogurt and granola make for a great breakfast indeed, but you need more than a snack-sized amount! Here you get creamy yogurt topped with fresh fruit and a generous amount of crunchy granola. Not only is this breakfast refreshing, but it's also satisfying. I like to use coconut-flavored yogurt or, for a vegan version, coconut milk yogurt, which is a consistent favorite of mine among all of the dairy-free yogurts I've tried.

While the homemade coconut-almond granola in this recipe is pretty darn tasty, please feel free to use store-bought granola to save time. Just look for one that would go with tropical flavors.

1 cup coconut-flavored yogurt or coconut milk yogurt

Peeled and sliced kiwi

Peeled and diced mango

Coconut-Almond Granola (recipe follows)

Scoop the yogurt into a bowl. Top with the kiwi, mango, and a handful or two of the granola. Serve immediately.

Coconut-Almond Granola

—— **MAKES** about 5 cups   **PREP TIME:** 15 minutes   **COOK TIME:** 40 minutes ——

2 tablespoons chia seeds

¼ cup plus 2 tablespoons water

⅓ cup pure maple syrup

3 tablespoons packed brown sugar

3 tablespoons coconut oil

½ teaspoon vanilla extract

¼ teaspoon almond extract

2 cups rolled oats

1 cup unsweetened shredded coconut

1 cup roughly chopped almonds

¼ cup hemp hearts

¼ teaspoon salt

1. Preheat the oven to 300°F. Line a sheet pan with parchment paper.

2. Mix the chia seeds and water in a small bowl. Set aside for 10 minutes to hydrate the seeds.

3. In a small saucepan over medium heat, whisk together the maple syrup, brown sugar, coconut oil, and extracts until the sugar dissolves. Remove from the heat.

4. In a large bowl, combine the oats, shredded coconut, almonds, hemp hearts, and salt. Stir in the maple syrup mixture and chia gel until well combined.

5. Spread the granola evenly on the parchment-lined pan. Bake for 20 minutes. Lightly push the granola around the edges toward the center, being careful not to break up too many clusters, and rotate the pan to help the granola bake evenly. Bake until the granola is crispy and golden, about 20 minutes longer.

6. Remove the pan from the oven and let the granola cool for at least 30 minutes. Break into pieces and store in a zip-top plastic bag or lidded container for up to 2 weeks.

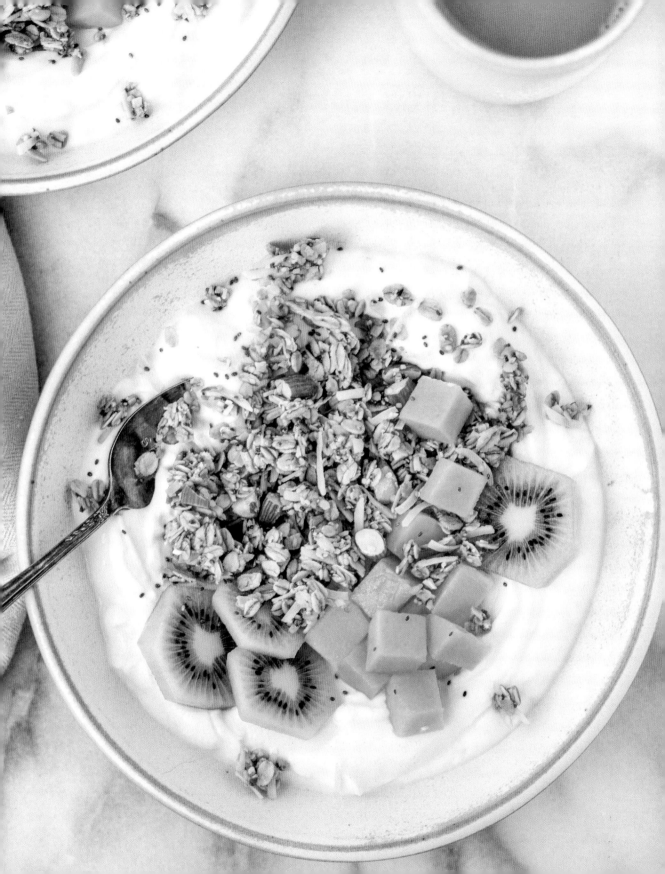

Peaches & Cream
OVERNIGHT OATS

—— MAKES 1 serving   PREP TIME: 10 minutes ——

Overnight oats are a fantastic option for a grab-and-go breakfast. Soaking rolled oats overnight in a mixture of yogurt and milk "cooks" and softens them into a creamy blend. I whip up individual servings in mason jars to top with fresh fruit, honey, and nuts or nut butter in the morning for a satisfying breakfast that takes just minutes. Meal prep isn't really my thing. However, with overnight oats being so simple and easy to throw together with just a few kitchen staples, it's not a hard habit to start.

A combination of yogurt and milk is essential in making the oats ultra-creamy and adding a dose of protein. The mashed banana adds subtle sweetness. Chia seeds, which gel up in liquid, add to the creamy texture while giving the end product a light crunch. Plus, they look pretty in there!

In South Carolina, the real peach state, we have access to the most perfect local peaches all summer long. They're bursting with juice, which I love to collect to drizzle over my oats. If you don't have fresh fruit on hand, top your oats with frozen fruit, thawed overnight in the fridge.

½ cup rolled oats

½ cup whole or 2% milk

¼ cup plain whole-milk or 2% Greek yogurt

½ banana, mashed

1½ teaspoons chia seeds

½ teaspoon vanilla extract

FOR SERVING:

Sliced ripe peaches

Honey

Hemp hearts

1. In a mason jar, mix together the oats, milk, yogurt, banana, chia seeds, and vanilla extract. Refrigerate overnight or for up to 5 days.

2. When ready to eat, top with peach slices, a drizzle of honey, and a sprinkle of hemp hearts.

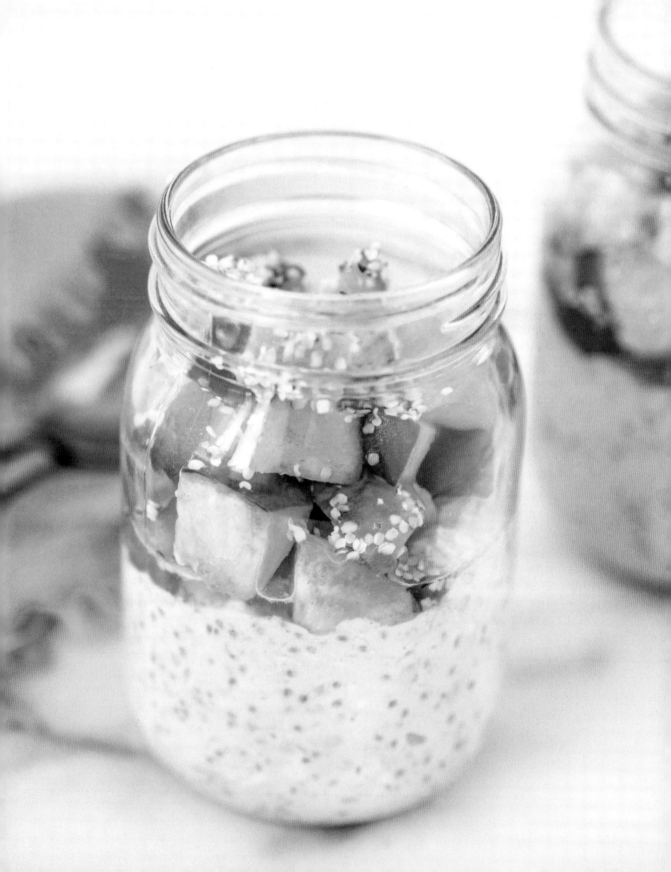

Sheet Pan Breakfast
BRUSSELS SPROUT HASH

———— MAKES 4 to 6 servings   PREP TIME: 10 minutes   COOK TIME: 40 minutes ————

Sheet pan meals are the ultimate when it comes to no-fuss meals with minimal cleanup. This recipe brings the sheet pan concept to breakfast with an easy and satisfying potato hash. Even though I call it a breakfast hash, I often make it for dinner as well. It's a pantry-friendly meal I never get sick of.

The trick to this hash lies in the use of bacon that renders its fat in the oven, flavoring the potatoes and Brussels sprouts (if you don't eat bacon, leave it out, or use vegan bacon). Crumbled chorizo will work as well. To switch it up and make this hash more interesting, I often use a mix of sweet potatoes and waxy white potatoes—usually fingerling or Yukon Gold.

Serve each portion of the hash topped with a fried or poached egg. Alternatively, you can cook the eggs all at once along with the hash by cracking them right on the hash about ten minutes before it's supposed to be done, then put the sheet pan back in the oven. When the hash turns golden brown, the eggs should be perfectly cooked, with the whites mostly set and the yolks still a little runny.

1½ pounds waxy potatoes, cut into ¾-inch cubes

2 cups Brussels sprouts, trimmed and halved

½ large yellow onion, diced

2 cloves garlic, minced

2 slices bacon, cut into ¼-inch pieces

1½ tablespoons extra-virgin olive oil, plus extra for frying the eggs

¼ teaspoon salt

¼ teaspoon cracked black pepper

4 to 6 large eggs

FOR SERVING:

Hot sauce

Thinly sliced scallions

Ketchup (optional)

1. Preheat the oven to 425°F.

2. In a large mixing bowl, toss the potatoes, Brussels sprouts, onion, garlic, and bacon until combined. Add the olive oil, salt, and pepper; toss again until every piece is thoroughly coated with the oil. Spread evenly on a sheet pan in a single layer.

3. Roast the hash for 20 minutes, stir, and continue to roast until golden brown and tender, about 20 minutes longer.

4. When the hash is almost finished, fry the eggs in olive oil as desired.

5. Divide the hash into 4 to 6 portions and serve each topped with a fried egg, hot sauce, and scallions, with ketchup on the side, if using.

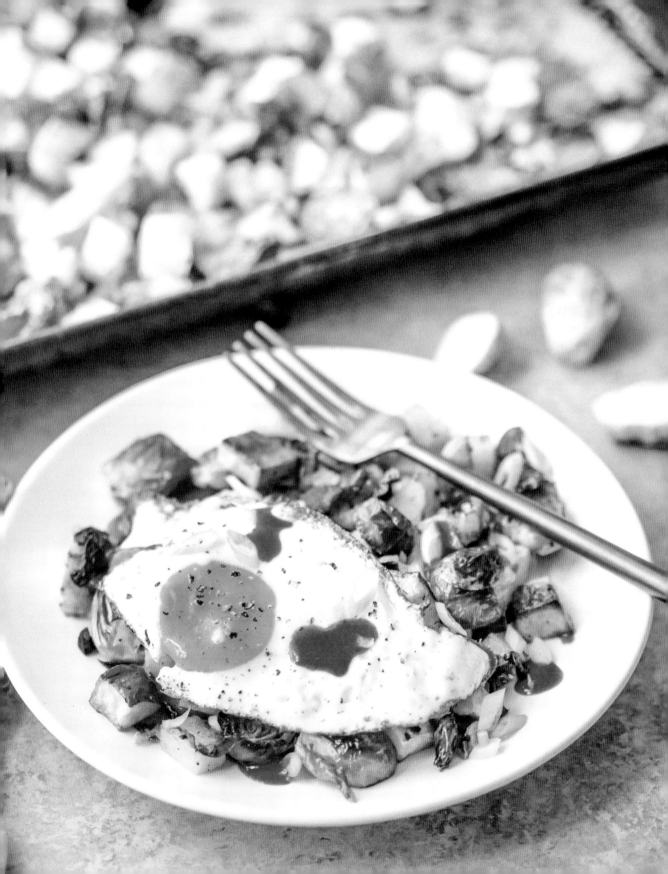

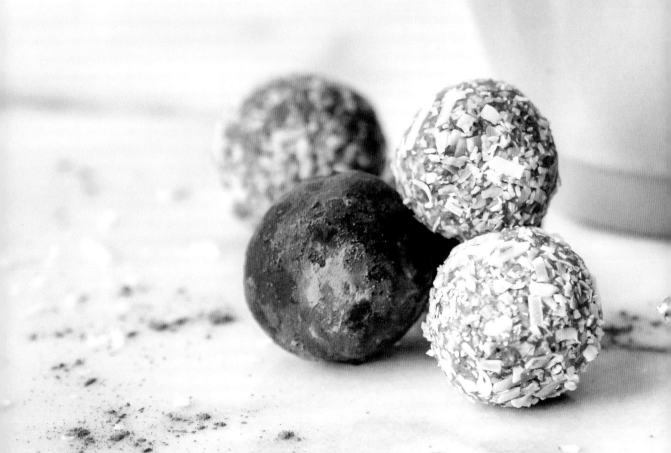

Chapter 8
SNACKS

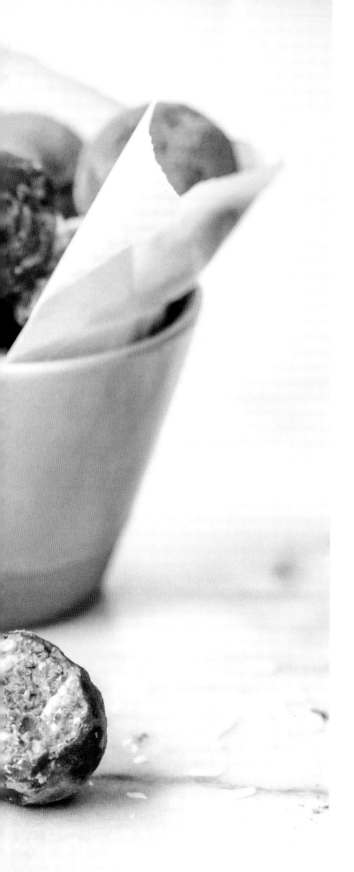

Savory Avocado & Cucumber
YOGURT BOWL

MAKES 1 serving   PREP TIME: 5 minutes

I've always loved the convenience of yogurt and granola as a packable snack. However, with my snacking preferences leaning toward savory, it's rarely a snack I'm in the mood for. So, when savory yogurt bowls became a trend a few years ago, I was fully on board! It makes a lot of sense since yogurt has traditionally been used in savory applications.

With creamy Greek yogurt and avocado, crisp and juicy cucumber, and crunchy roasted chickpeas, this savory yogurt bowl has got tons of fun textures going on. Packed with fats and protein, it's also both filling and satisfying. To turn it into a light meal, you can add to it halved cherry tomatoes, sliced Kalamata olives, and crumbled feta cheese and serve it with pita chips.

If you want to make this bowl in advance, sprinkling the avocado with lemon juice will prevent it from browning for at least a day.

½ to ¾ cup plain whole-milk or 2% Greek yogurt

¼ avocado, diced

¼ cup diced cucumbers

Extra-virgin olive oil

Lemon juice

Grated lemon zest

Store-bought roasted chickpea snacks

Chopped herbs, such as mint, dill, and/or basil

Flaky sea salt

Put the yogurt in a bowl and make a well in the center with the back of a spoon. Fill the well with the avocado and cucumber. Drizzle with some olive oil, a spritz of lemon juice, and a sprinkle of lemon zest. Garnish with a handful of roasted chickpeas, some fresh herbs, and a pinch of flaky salt.

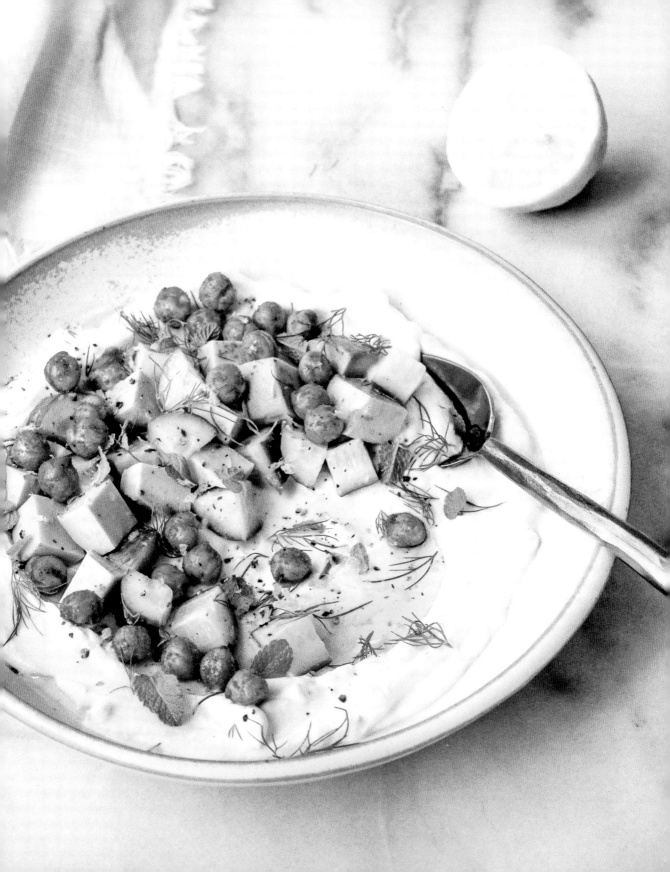

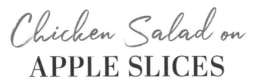

Chicken Salad on
APPLE SLICES

MAKES 4 cups chicken salad (4 to 6 servings)   PREP TIME: 15 minutes

Chicken or tuna salad and crackers is one of my all-time favorite satisfying snacks. One day, I found myself with a big tub of chicken salad but no crackers for snacking. So I came up with what I thought was an ingenious idea of turning apples into crackers by cutting them into rounds and cutting out the seeds in the center. If you love the sweet kick of apples or grapes in your chicken salad, you'll love using fruit as a vehicle for chicken salad!

I like to make my chicken salad with a mixture of half mayonnaise and half plain whole-milk Greek yogurt. I love the tang of Greek yogurt, which, along with the lemon zest, gives the salad a fresher taste. Some "healthy" chicken salad recipes use only yogurt for dressing, but it's mayonnaise that adds the essential flavor. Mayonnaise is nothing to be afraid of. Diet culture tends to push oil and vinegar dressings over creamy mayo-based dressings, but what some perhaps fail to recognize is that mayonnaise literally is oil and vinegar emulsified with a bit of egg!

For a vegetarian version, replace the chicken salad with the herbed chickpea salad on page 186.

3 cups shredded rotisserie chicken

1 celery stalk, diced

3 tablespoons roughly chopped toasted almonds

2 tablespoons minced shallots

1 tablespoon finely chopped parsley

Grated zest of 1 lemon

¼ cup plain whole-milk or 2% Greek yogurt

¼ cup mayonnaise

2 teaspoons whole-grain mustard

Salt and black pepper

4 medium apples, for serving

1. Put the chicken, celery, almonds, shallots, parsley, and lemon zest in a large bowl. Add the yogurt, mayonnaise, and mustard; stir to combine. Season with salt and pepper to taste.

2. Slice the apples crosswise into thin rounds. Remove the seeds. Top each round with a spoonful of chicken salad and enjoy.

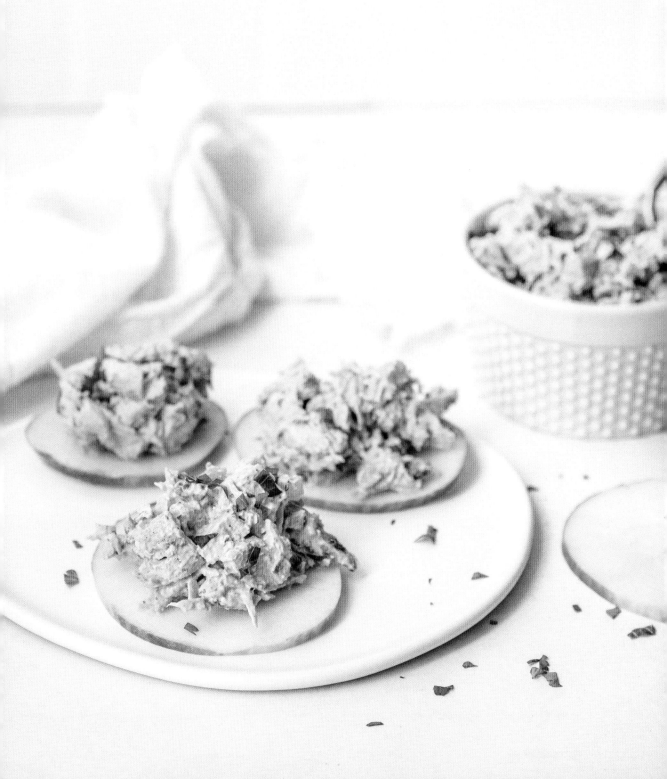

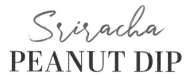

Sriracha
PEANUT DIP

MAKES 2 cups (4 servings)   PREP TIME: 5 minutes

Based on my observation, diet culture's propensity to label food as "good" or "bad" is never more obvious than in the realm of snacks. It deems potato chips, cookies, or crackers "bad," and fresh fruits or raw veggies with dip (usually the obligatory low-fat ranch dressing) "good." Such labeling not only makes it hard for people to eat the "bad" foods without a side of guilt, but it can also ruin the "good" foods by turning them into a chore.

The key is to make vegetables part of a satisfying snack, and not to use them as a stomach filler. Rounds of crisp cucumber are the perfect accompaniment to this spicy Sriracha peanut dip. That said, I find rice crackers—with their crunch and satisfaction factor—to work well here also.

Made with a blend of chickpeas and peanut butter and seasoned with lime juice, Sriracha, ginger, and soy sauce, this dip has a flavor reminiscent of a Southeast Asian peanut sauce. It will keep for about a week in the fridge.

1 (15-ounce) can chickpeas, drained and rinsed

¼ cup creamy peanut butter

2 tablespoons fresh lime juice

1 tablespoon soy sauce

1 clove garlic, minced

2 to 3 teaspoons Sriracha sauce, plus extra for drizzling

2 teaspoons grated ginger

1 teaspoon honey

¼ cup peanut oil

Salt

FOR GARNISH:

Chopped toasted peanuts

Thinly sliced scallions

Chopped cilantro

1. In a food processor, blend the chickpeas, peanut butter, lime juice, soy sauce, garlic, Sriracha, ginger, and honey until well combined. With the motor running, pour in the peanut oil in a thin stream. Blend, scraping down the sides as needed, until creamy and smooth, about 2 minutes. Season with salt to taste.

2. Serve the dip drizzled with Sriracha and garnished with peanuts, scallions, and cilantro.

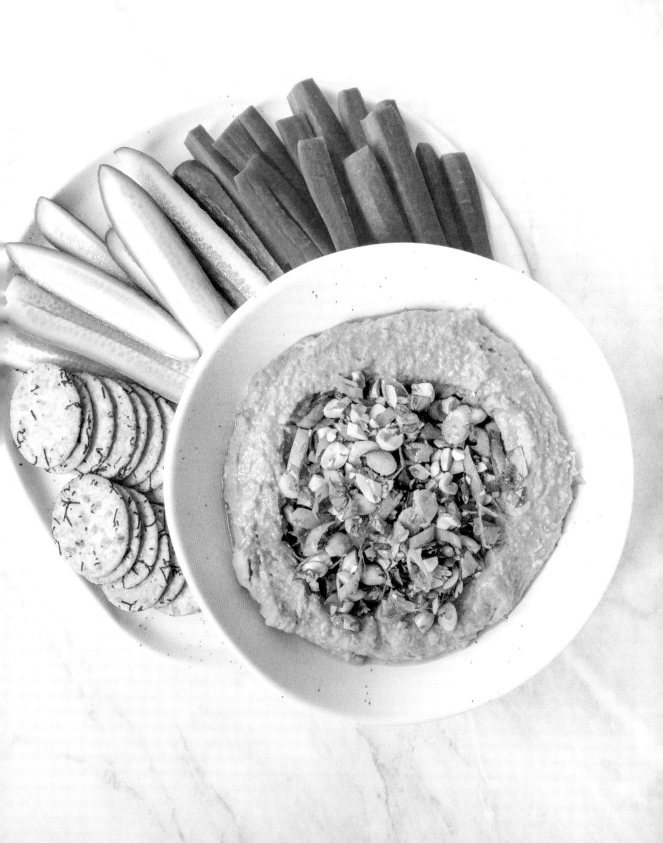

Trail Mix
THREE WAYS

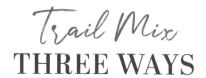

MAKES amount desired   PREP TIME: 5 minutes

Trail mix is a satisfying snack, but if you're anything like me, you probably tire of the same old blends sold at the grocery store. Get creative with whatever pantry staples you have on hand! When I make homemade trail mix, I like to put it in individual baggies or mini mason jars so I can grab one and throw it in my purse for a portable snack. To make these mixes, I generally like to combine equal quantities of each ingredient, but feel free to add more or less of the ingredients you love. Because I have left out specific measurements, you can quickly throw together a single serving or make a large enough batch to last a week or two.

SALTY BANANA–PEANUT BUTTER MIX:

1 part pretzels

1 part salted roasted peanuts

1 part peanut butter chips or candies

1 part banana chips

TROPICAL SPICY MANGO MIX:

1 part raw almonds

1 part dried chili mango slices

1 part dried coconut chips or flakes

CHOCOLATE-CHERRY MIX:

1 part raw walnuts

1 part raw or roasted shelled pistachios

1 part raw pumpkin seeds

1 part semisweet chocolate chunks

1 part dried cherries

Put the ingredients for the mix of your choice in a large zip-top plastic bag or lidded container and shake to combine.

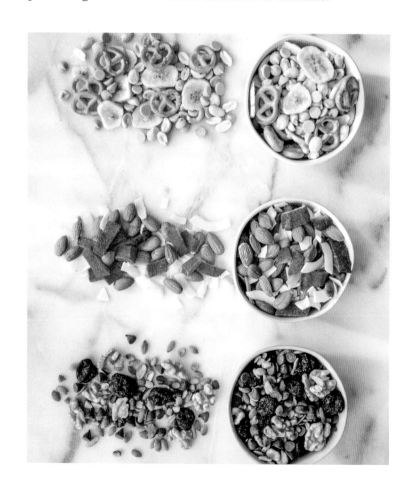

Crunchy Honey–Almond
ENERGY BITES

MAKES about 20 bites   PREP TIME: 15 minutes

One mistake that's sure to make you hate working out is trying to exercise with no fuel in your body. When you're moving for fun and not for calorie burning, it makes a lot more sense to fuel your body properly! These honey-almond bites are packed with energy, and they will fuel your workout without leaving you with an overly full stomach. They are also great for those times when you need a quick burst of glucose to carry you through to your next meal.

½ cup rolled oats

1¼ cups salted almond butter

¼ cup honey

2 cups puffed brown rice

Cocoa powder and/or shredded coconut, for coating

1.   Pulse the oats in a food processor until coarsely ground. Add the almond butter and honey and blend until combined. Add the puffed brown rice and pulse until combined, scraping down the sides as needed.

2.   Using your hands, roll the mixture into golf ball–sized bites. Roll each ball in cocoa powder or shredded coconut. Refrigerate for up to 2 weeks.

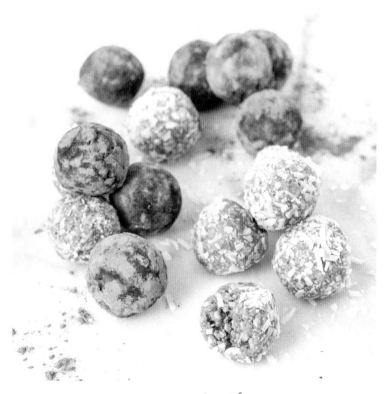

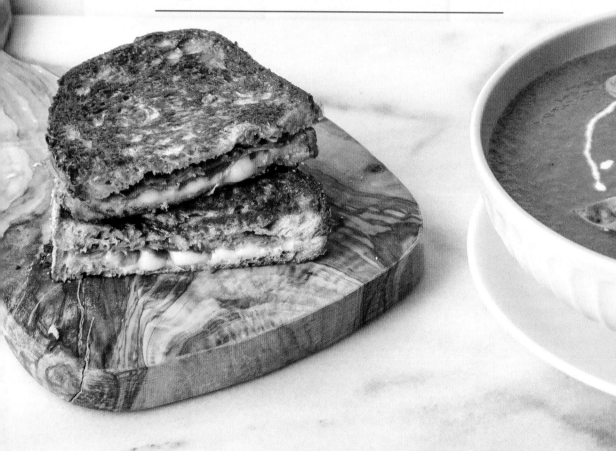

Chapter 9
SOUPS
& SALADS

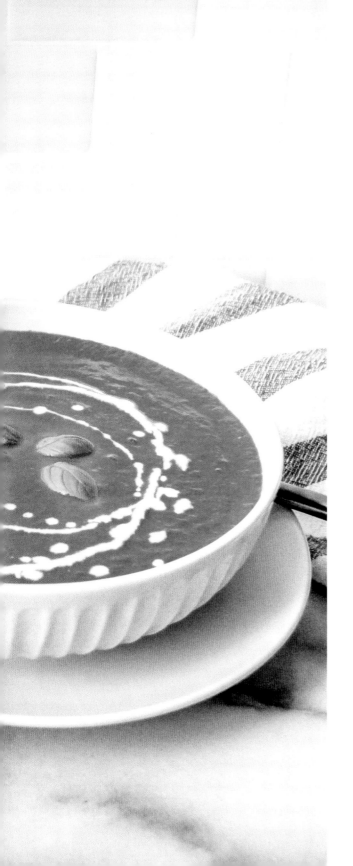

Broccoli, White Bean & CHEDDAR SOUP

MAKES 4 servings **PREP TIME: 20 minutes** **COOK TIME: 15 minutes**

Is there anything more comforting than a creamy, cheesy bowl of soup? This broccoli and cheddar soup gets a boost of protein from canned cannellini beans, which also help thicken the soup. It's a simple trick you can use to add satisfying protein to almost any puréed vegetable soup recipe.

This recipe uses an immersion blender to purée the soup in the pot. It's an inexpensive piece of equipment that doesn't take up much room in the kitchen and makes preparing puréed soups a breeze! If you don't have an immersion blender, carefully purée the soup in batches in a regular countertop blender. If you like chunks of broccoli in your soup, pull out a couple pieces and add them back to the soup after blending. Also, if you like your soup on the thicker side, make it with three cups of broth and stir in the remaining 1 cup of the broth at the end, a little at a time, until it reaches desired consistency.

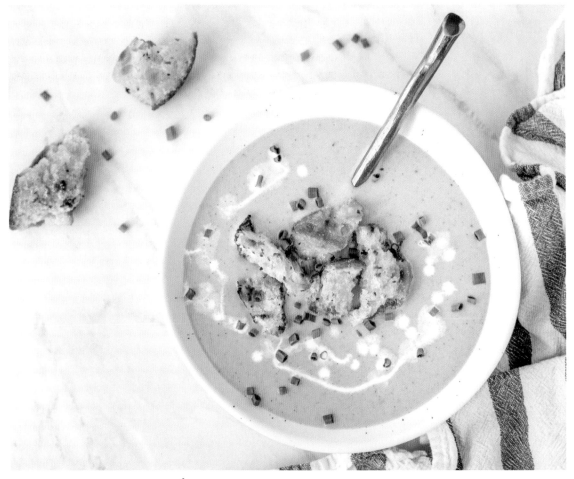

SOUP:

2 tablespoons extra-virgin olive oil

½ large yellow onion, roughly chopped

4 cloves garlic, lightly crushed

1 large carrot, roughly chopped

½ teaspoon dried thyme

⅛ teaspoon ground nutmeg

Pinch of cayenne pepper

4 cups low-sodium chicken or vegetable broth

1 head broccoli, stem included, roughly chopped

1 (15.5-ounce) can cannellini beans, drained and rinsed

½ teaspoon salt

¼ teaspoon cracked black pepper

1 cup shredded sharp cheddar cheese, plus extra for topping if desired

1 cup whole milk or half-and-half, plus extra for drizzling if desired

1 teaspoon whole-grain mustard

CIABATTA CROUTONS:

2 tablespoons extra-virgin olive oil

2½ cups bite-sized torn ciabatta bread

¼ teaspoon garlic powder

1. Heat the olive oil in a large saucepan over medium-high heat. Add the onion, garlic, and carrot and sauté until the onion is translucent, about 5 minutes. Stir in the thyme, nutmeg, and cayenne and cook until fragrant, about 1 minute.

2. Add the broth, broccoli, beans, salt, and black pepper. Bring to a boil, reduce the heat, and simmer, partially covered, until the broccoli is tender, about 10 minutes.

3. While the soup is simmering, make the croutons: Heat the olive oil in a large skillet over medium heat. Add the torn ciabatta and toast, stirring frequently, until golden brown and crispy, about 5 minutes. Turn off the heat and immediately sprinkle with the garlic powder.

4. When the soup is done, turn off the heat and use an immersion blender to purée the soup. Add the cheese, milk, and mustard; stir until the cheese melts. Season with more salt and black pepper to taste. Serve topped with the croutons and some extra cheddar or a drizzle of milk, if desired.

Roasted Tomato–Basil Soup
WITH PROSCIUTTO & PESTO GRILLED CHEESE

MAKES 6 to 8 servings of soup, plus desired number of sandwiches   PREP TIME: 30 minutes

—— COOK TIME: 24 minutes ——

This recipe is an attempt to make up for my first—and perhaps most epic—cooking fail. I was a junior in college and had just moved into my first apartment. After two years of dining hall meals, I was beyond thrilled to have access to a kitchen. But instead of starting off easy, I got a little overly excited and picked out a bunch of complicated and fussy recipes to break in my kitchen, not realizing just how much time and how many ingredients were involved.

One night before an important meeting, I decided to try my hand at making a roasted tomato soup served with smoked-mozzarella grilled cheese. Mistake number one was picking a new recipe to cook on a time crunch! Mistake number two was, in my flustered state, rushing to make it to my meeting on time, putting my beautiful tomato soup, complete with actual roasted tomatoes, into my cheap blender to purée. When I hit blend, boiling hot and bright red tomato soup exploded out of the blender! It ended up all over my clothes and in my hair, coating our entire kitchen, including the ceiling. My roommates were not too pleased!

This is a simpler version of that recipe. Instead of vegetables roasted from scratch, it calls for canned fire-roasted tomatoes, which impart a slightly smoky flavor to the soup. Since that messy incident, I've learned that an immersion blender, as I explained earlier (see page 168), is useful for making a puréed soup. If you've got a panini press, you'll want to break it out for the grilled cheese sandwiches also.

SOUP:

2 tablespoons extra-virgin olive oil

1 large yellow onion, roughly chopped

1 large carrot, roughly chopped

6 cloves garlic, minced

Salt and black pepper

2 tablespoons tomato paste

⅛ to ¼ teaspoon red pepper flakes, depending on heat preference

1 (28-ounce) can fire-roasted tomatoes

1. Heat the olive oil in a large saucepan over medium-high heat. Add the onion, carrot, and garlic along with a pinch of salt and pepper. Sauté until the onion is lightly golden and the carrot is tender, about 7 minutes.

2. Stir in the tomato paste and red pepper flakes and cook for 1 to 2 minutes. Stir in the tomatoes, broth, and bay leaf. Bring to a boil, reduce the heat, and simmer for 10 to 15 minutes to let the flavors meld.

3. Meanwhile, prepare the sandwiches. To make one sandwich, spread the pesto on one slice of bread. Top with the mozzarella and prosciutto, then the other slice of bread. Melt a small pat of butter in a medium skillet over medium heat. Place the sandwich in the skillet and cook, pressing down with the back of a spatula, until the cheese melts and the bread turns golden and crispy, about 2 minutes per side.

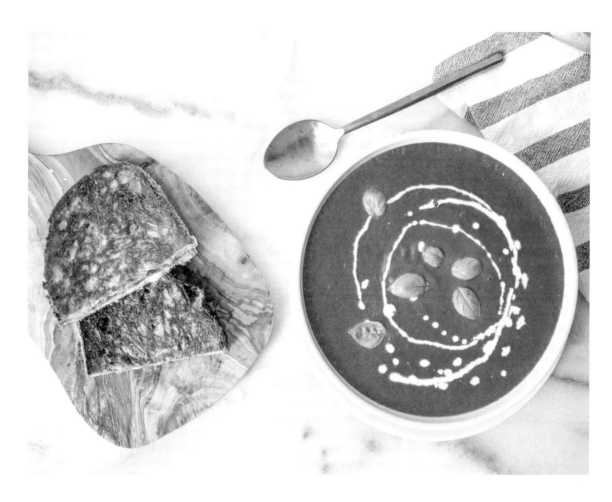

3 cups low-sodium chicken or vegetable broth

1 bay leaf

¼ cup basil leaves

Heavy cream, crème fraîche, or mascarpone, for serving

SANDWICHES (PER SANDWICH):

2 slices bread, preferably sourdough

1 to 2 tablespoons pesto

⅓ to ½ cup shredded mozzarella cheese

1 or 2 thin slices prosciutto

Butter

4. Remove the bay leaf from the soup and discard it. Stir in the basil leaves and carefully blend the soup with an immersion blender or in a countertop blender until creamy. Season with more salt and black pepper to taste. Top with a drizzle of cream or a small spoonful of crème fraîche or mascarpone and serve alongside the grilled cheese sandwich.

Easy
DUMPLING SOUP

MAKES 2 to 4 servings PREP TIME: 10 minutes COOK TIME: 12 minutes

Dumplings are among my all-time favorite comfort foods. After a particularly rough day, if my husband is out of town, I've been known to pan-fry a bunch of frozen dumplings and eat them for dinner with soy and chili sauce while in bed watching Netflix. Now you know my comfort eating secrets! However, when I have the energy, using dumplings in a meal rather than as my meal is a little more satisfying.

This easy dumpling soup is my way of turning store-bought frozen dumplings into a full-on meal that's both balanced and filling, with the addition of shiitake mushrooms and baby spinach to round it out. If you want to make it even heartier, serve it over steamed rice.

1 tablespoon toasted sesame oil

2 ounces fresh shiitake mushrooms, thinly sliced

Pinch of salt

2 scallions, sliced

1 tablespoon minced ginger

2 cloves garlic, minced

6 cups low-sodium chicken or vegetable broth

1 pound frozen wontons or gyoza dumplings

2 handfuls fresh baby spinach (about 2 ounces)

1 to 2 tablespoons soy sauce

FOR SERVING (OPTIONAL):

Sriracha sauce

Fresh lemon or lime juice

1. Heat the sesame oil in a large saucepan over medium-high heat. Add the mushrooms and salt and cook, stirring occasionally, until golden, about 5 minutes. Stir in the scallions, ginger, and garlic and cook until fragrant, about 1 minute.

2. Pour in the broth, cover, and bring to a boil. When the broth reaches a rolling boil, drop in the frozen wontons. Bring to a simmer and cook for 3 to 5 minutes, or according to the package instructions.

3. Stir in the spinach, cover, and cook until wilted, about 30 seconds. Season to taste with the soy sauce.

4. Divide the soup among 2 to 4 bowls. If desired, serve with Sriracha and lemon or lime juice.

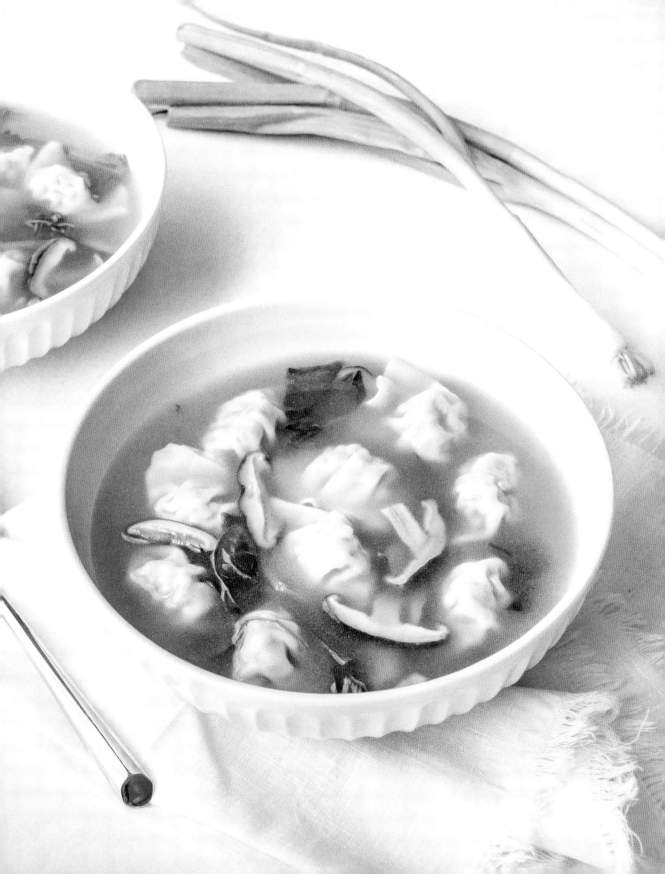

The Best
VEGETARIAN CHILI

MAKES 6 to 8 servings PREP TIME: 20 minutes COOK TIME: 1 hour

Canned chili is a staple in my house for making easy lunches of chili-stuffed baked sweet potatoes and chili cheese fries and rounding out easy salads to make a meal. However, nothing beats homemade chili. When I make it, I like to break out my biggest saucepan, double the recipe, and freeze the leftovers. I've had my fair share of vegetarian chili, and this hearty recipe, with a mixture of beans and tons of veggies, is my absolute favorite. It is sure to become your go-to.

Store the leftover chipotle chilies in the freezer and pull out a couple as needed for soups, stews, marinades, or salsas.

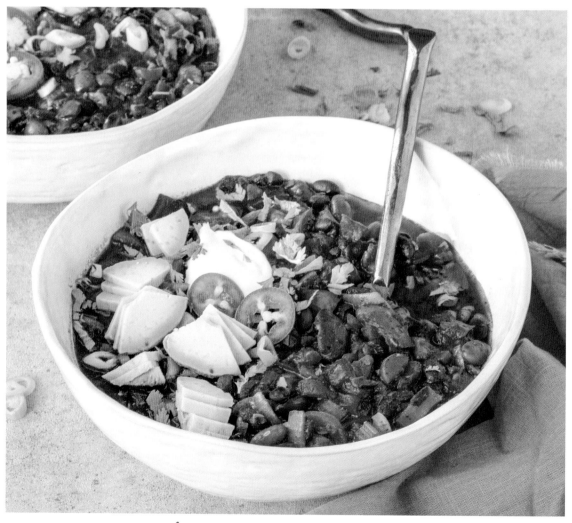

2 tablespoons extra-virgin olive oil

1 large yellow onion, diced

2 large carrots, diced

2 celery stalks, diced

1 red bell pepper, deseeded and diced

1 jalapeño pepper, deseeded and finely diced

½ teaspoon plus a pinch of salt, divided

8 ounces cremini mushrooms, diced

6 cloves garlic, minced

2 tablespoons tomato paste

2 chipotle chilies, minced, from a can of chipotle chilis in adobo sauce

2 tablespoons chili powder

2 teaspoons ground cumin

2 teaspoons unsweetened cocoa powder

1 teaspoon dried oregano

1 bay leaf

2 cups low-sodium vegetable broth

2 (15-ounce) cans fire-roasted diced tomatoes

1 (15-ounce) can black beans, drained and rinsed

1 (15-ounce) can kidney beans, drained and rinsed

1 (15-ounce) can pinto beans, drained and rinsed

¼ teaspoon cracked black pepper

OPTIONAL GARNISHES:

Sliced avocado

Chopped cilantro

Thinly sliced scallions

Sour cream or plain whole-milk or 2% Greek yogurt

Sliced jalapeño peppers

1. Heat the olive oil in a 6- or 7-quart Dutch oven over medium-high heat. Add the onion, carrots, celery, bell pepper, jalapeño, and a pinch of salt. Cook until the onion is translucent, 7 to 10 minutes. Stir in the mushrooms and garlic and cook until the mushrooms are tender, 5 to 7 minutes.

2. Add the tomato paste, chipotles, chili powder, cumin, cocoa powder, oregano, and bay leaf; cook, stirring constantly, until fragrant, about 1 minute.

3. Pour in the broth, stirring up any browned bits at the bottom of the pot. Stir in the tomatoes, beans, salt, and pepper and bring to a boil. Partially cover, reduce the heat to medium, and simmer until thickened, 30 to 40 minutes.

4. Remove and discard the bay leaf. Season with more salt and pepper to taste. Serve in bowls, garnished as desired.

Kale Salad with Chicken,
ROASTED SQUASH &
MAPLE-DIJON VINAIGRETTE

MAKES 2 to 3 servings   PREP TIME: 20 minutes   COOK TIME: 35 minutes

News flash: salads don't have to suck! This may be the most dietitian-y thing I will say in this book, but the food I am saddest about diet culture ruining is the salad. Recipes like this are a reminder that salads can be so much more than a sad bed of greens and bland, dried-out chicken breast.

A satisfying salad has to begin with flavorful greens, like baby kale, which is tender yet earthy with a slight bitterness. It also needs a flavorful protein; in this recipe, I use tender and juicy rotisserie chicken as a shortcut. Then it should have a carbohydrate source; the caramelized butternut squash in this recipe plays this role while lending its cozy flavor. Also, a salad needs flavor boosters; it's hard to go wrong with a flavorful cheese, toasted nuts, and crispy bacon—all of which we have here. Last but not least, a truly satisfying salad needs a killer dressing. While there are plenty of really tasty store-bought options, I love the bright and fresh taste of this maple-Dijon vinaigrette, which calls for pantry staples and takes just a couple of minutes to whip up.

1 medium butternut squash, peeled, deseeded, and cut into 1-inch cubes (about 3 cups)

1 tablespoon extra-virgin olive oil

Salt and black pepper

⅓ cup raw walnuts

4 slices bacon

1 (5-ounce) bag baby kale

Desired amount of rotisserie chicken meat, chopped into bite-sized pieces

⅓ cup crumbled goat cheese

MAPLE-DIJON VINAIGRETTE:

¼ cup walnut oil or extra-virgin olive oil

2 tablespoons apple cider vinegar

2 tablespoons maple syrup

1 tablespoon Dijon mustard

Salt and black pepper

1.   Preheat the oven to 400°F.

2.   Toss the squash cubes with the olive oil and a pinch of salt and pepper and spread evenly on a sheet pan. Roast, stirring halfway through cooking, until tender and golden, 30 to 35 minutes.

3.   Meanwhile, prepare the vinaigrette: Put the walnut oil, vinegar, maple syrup, and mustard in a mason jar and shake to combine. Season with salt and pepper to taste and shake again.

4.   Toast the walnuts in a medium skillet over medium heat, stirring frequently, until fragrant, 2 to 3 minutes. Remove from the skillet and wipe the pan clean.

5.   Add the bacon to the skillet and cook until crispy, flipping the slices over halfway through cooking, about 7 minutes. Remove to a paper towel–lined plate. When cool enough to handle, crumble the bacon.

6.   Toss the kale with the vinaigrette. Divide between 2 or 3 plates. Top with the squash, chicken, walnuts, bacon, and goat cheese and serve.

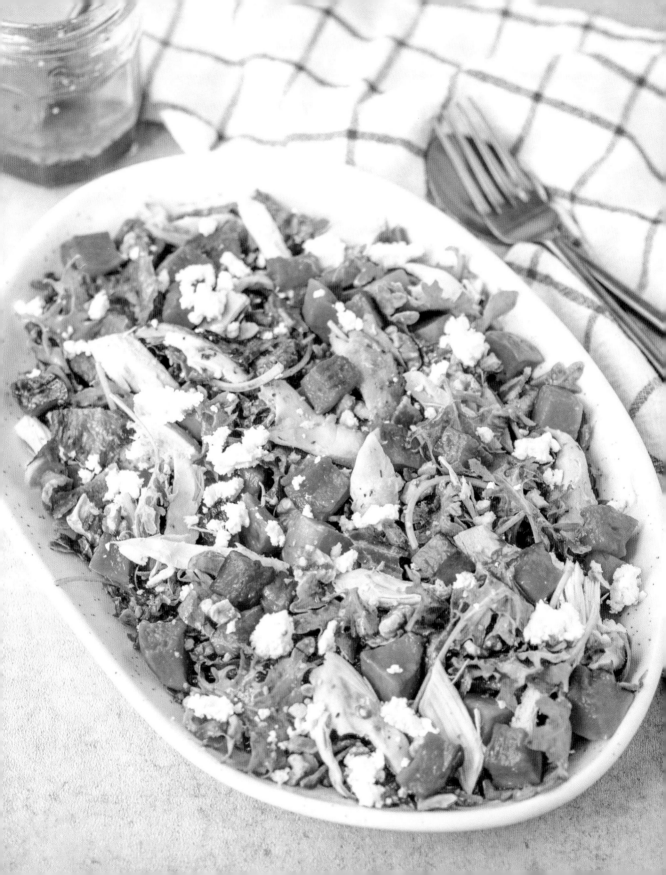

California Salad with Crispy Baked
TOFU & PEANUT DRESSING

MAKES 3 to 4 servings   PREP TIME: 20 minutes   COOK TIME: 35 minutes

If you think you don't like tofu, just wait until you try the crispy baked tofu in this recipe. I promise it will convert you! It was inspired by the house tofu at Papas and Pollo in Sonoma, a favorite restaurant of my sister and brother-in-law, who live nearby. When a thirty-something-year-old welder tells you that the tofu is his favorite thing on the menu, you listen! Though the folks at the restaurant didn't give me the recipe, they did tell me that nutritional yeast was the secret ingredient, so I was able to hack my own version from there. I serve this tofu in tacos, over grain bowls, and in salads, like this fresh and crunchy salad with peanut dressing.

Nutritional yeast, sometimes referred to as "nooch," is standard in vegan kitchens. By itself, I don't think it tastes very good, but it adds a pleasant, cheesy flavor when mixed into sauces or sprinkled into dishes. When stored in a jar in a cool dark place, it will last for up to two years.

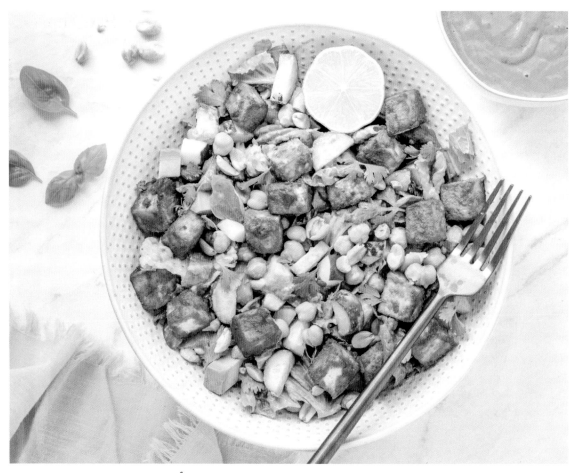

CRISPY BAKED TOFU:

1 (16-ounce) block extra-firm tofu, pressed to remove liquid

¼ cup nutritional yeast

3 tablespoons soy sauce

1 tablespoon extra-virgin olive oil

½ teaspoon ground cumin

¼ teaspoon garlic powder

PEANUT DRESSING:

¼ cup creamy peanut butter

Juice of 1 lime

1 small shallot, chopped

1 clove garlic, peeled

2 tablespoons minced ginger

2 tablespoons peanut oil or toasted sesame oil

2 tablespoons soy sauce

1 tablespoon granulated sugar

Salt

SALAD:

1 heart of romaine, chopped, rinsed, and spun dry

1 cup thinly sliced napa cabbage, rinsed and spun dry

1 (15-ounce) can chickpeas, drained and rinsed

1 avocado, halved, pitted, cut into ½-inch cubes

3 radishes, cut into ½-inch cubes

½ large cucumber or 2 Persian cucumbers, sliced into ¼-inch-thick half-moons

¼ cup loosely packed basil leaves, roughly chopped if large

¼ cup loosely packed cilantro leaves

¼ cup loosely packed mint leaves

⅓ cup roasted peanuts

1. Preheat the oven to 400°F. Line a sheet pan with parchment paper.

2. Cut the tofu into ¾-inch cubes. In a large bowl, whisk together the nutritional yeast, soy sauce, olive oil, cumin, and garlic powder. Stir in the tofu; toss until thoroughly coated. Set aside to marinate for at least 15 minutes.

3. While the tofu is marinating, prepare the dressing: Put the peanut butter, lime juice, shallot, garlic, ginger, peanut oil, soy sauce, and sugar in a food processor or blender and blend until creamy, scraping down the sides as needed. Season with salt to taste.

4. Remove the tofu from the marinade and spread it evenly on the prepared sheet pan. Bake, tossing the cubes halfway through cooking, until crispy on the outside, about 35 minutes.

5. Toss the romaine, cabbage, chickpeas, avocado, radishes, cucumber, and herbs together in a large bowl. Add the dressing and toss to combine.

6. Divide the salad among 3 or 4 bowls. Top with the tofu and peanuts before serving.

Meal Prep Cilantro-Lime
CHICKEN SALAD (OR GRAIN BOWL)

———————— MAKES 3 or 4 salads/bowls PREP TIME: 30 minutes COOK TIME: 15 minutes ————————

I have a bit of a love-hate relationship with meal prep. While the color-coordinated, perfectly portioned containers can be a bit intimidating, I know that for many people, meal prep is essential to getting fed while staying sane during the week.

If you're tired of your usual lunch salad, or you've had a few too many of those standard-issue chicken, broccoli, and brown rice meal preps, you'll love this cilantro-lime chicken salad. It's fresh, flavorful, and packed with nourishing ingredients to power you through the afternoon. Depending on your hunger level, you can serve this as a salad or grain bowl style! Just prep and pack the toppings separately and scoop them over a bed of cooked quinoa or salad greens. Look for frozen quinoa at the grocery store, which allows you to make a game-time decision without having to boil water.

CHICKEN:

⅓ cup extra-virgin olive oil

⅓ cup fresh lime juice

⅓ cup chopped cilantro

2 teaspoons honey

2 cloves garlic, minced

Salt and black pepper

1½ pounds boneless, skinless chicken breasts

SALAD:

2 ears corn, husks removed

1 to 2 teaspoons extra-virgin olive oil

Salt and black pepper

Salad greens or cooked quinoa

1 (15-ounce) can black beans, drained and rinsed

1 cup halved cherry tomatoes

½ large cucumber or 2 Persian cucumbers, deseeded and thinly sliced crosswise

⅓ cup crumbled goat cheese

1. Marinate the chicken: Whisk together the olive oil, lime juice, cilantro, honey, and garlic and season with salt and pepper. Place the chicken in a mixing bowl and toss with ¼ cup of the marinade, reserving the remainder for use as a dressing. Refrigerate the chicken for at least 30 minutes or up to 8 hours.

2. When ready to cook the chicken, heat a gas grill to medium-high heat. (If using a charcoal grill, light half a chimney of coals, wait until the coals are covered in a faint coating of white ash, and spread them on the bottom grate.) Rub the corn with the olive oil and season with salt and pepper. Place the chicken in a large zip-top plastic bag, seal, and whack a few times with a meat mallet to flatten the breasts slightly. This will help the chicken cook faster and more evenly while also tenderizing it a bit.

3. Grill the chicken until cooked through and grill-marked on both sides, 5 to 7 minutes per side. Grill the corn, turning every few minutes, until lightly charred, about 10 minutes. Remove the chicken and corn to a plate and set aside to cool slightly.

4. Meanwhile, divide the greens or quinoa among 3 or 4 salad bowls or portable containers. Top with the black beans, tomatoes, cucumber, and goat cheese, or, if prepping for later, place these ingredients in a separate portable container.

5. Use a serrated knife to slice the corn kernels off the cob. Slice the chicken on the diagonal. Divide the corn and chicken among the salads (or add to the container of toppings). Just before eating, drizzle each salad with the reserved dressing.

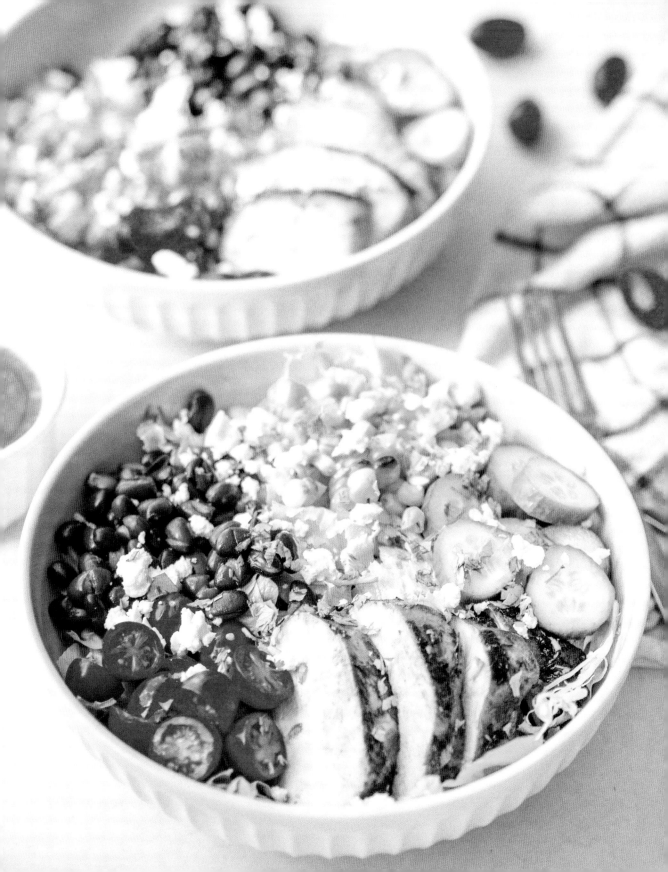

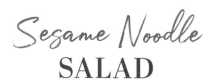

Sesame Noodle
SALAD

MAKES 3 to 4 servings   PREP TIME: 5 minutes   COOK TIME: 10 minutes

When you want the fresh taste of a salad but the satisfaction of carbs, look to noodle salad. Served cool with tons of crunchy, hydrating vegetables, this noodle salad is on heavy rotation for me in the summer. I like to use dried soba or dried rice sticks (aka pad thai noodles), but good old spaghetti will work in a pinch. Feel free to use peanut butter in place of the tahini to make peanut noodle salad. (If you go with the peanut version, add some fresh mango to this salad to take it to the next level.) To round out this meal with The Gang, serve it topped with your choice of protein, such as cooked chicken, grilled shrimp, diced baked tofu, or pan-fried dumplings.

8 ounces dried soba noodles or dried rice sticks

¼ cup plus 1 tablespoon tahini

2 tablespoons toasted sesame oil

2 tablespoons soy sauce

1 tablespoon packed brown sugar

1 tablespoon unseasoned rice vinegar

2 teaspoons Sriracha sauce

2 carrots, peeled and grated on the large holes of a cheese grater

1 large cucumber, sliced into ¼-inch-thick half-moons

½ cup thinly sliced scallions

2 tablespoons chopped cilantro

Chopped or torn butter lettuce, for serving (optional)

1. Cook the soba noodles according to the package instructions. Drain and rinse with cold water.

2. While the noodles are cooking, make the dressing: Whisk together the tahini, sesame oil, soy sauce, brown sugar, rice vinegar, and Sriracha.

3. Toss the noodles with the dressing until well combined. Add the carrots, cucumber, scallions, and cilantro and toss again. If desired, serve over a bed of butter lettuce.

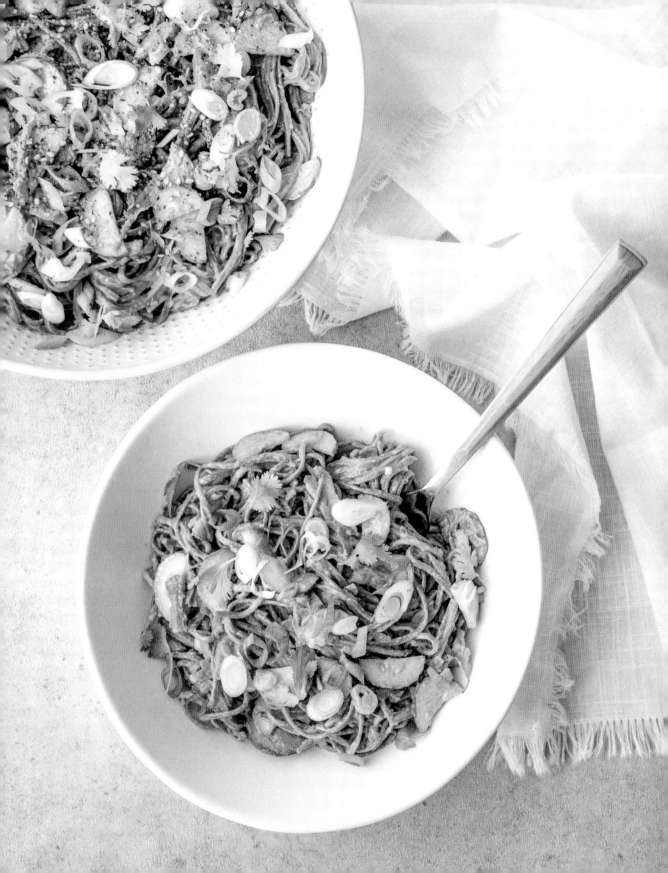

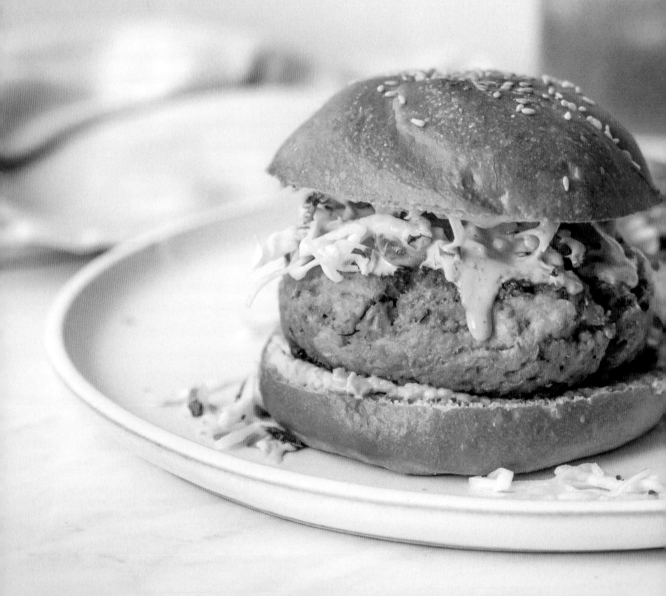

Chapter 10
MAIN DISHES

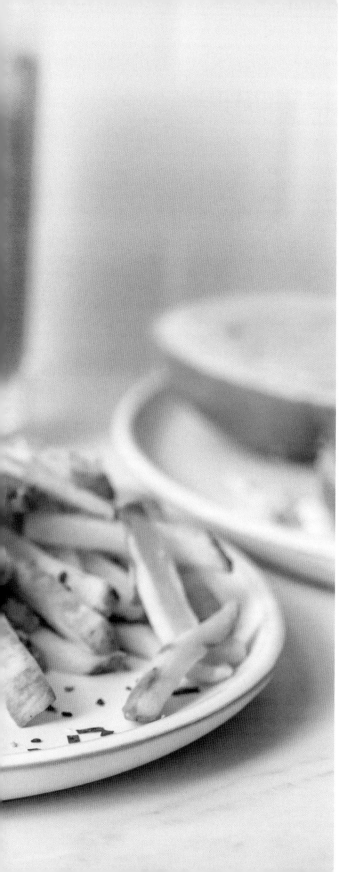

Herbed Chickpea
SALAD SANDWICHES

MAKES 3 or 4 sandwiches   PREP TIME: 15 minutes

When I was in middle school, I decided to become a vegetarian. My best friend was doing it, and thus so was I! I said I was doing it for the animals, but—who were we kidding?—I just thought it made me sound cool. Although that period of my life involved a fair number of microwaved frozen veggie burgers, I still managed to eat pretty good food thanks to my parents, both of whom were pretty creative cooks. The one sad spot in my meals? My lunchtime sandwiches. I ate peanut butter and jelly almost exclusively for nearly two years because what else are you going to do? I wish I could go back in time and tell middle school Rachael that a) dressing like a Spice Girl is not cool, b) you shouldn't cut out entire food groups based on what your best friend is doing, and c) if you refuse to listen to future Rachael regarding food groups, at least pack this herbed chickpea salad sandwich.

This recipe was a favorite among my taste-testers (aka my husband, my family, and my friends). If you're looking to incorporate more meatless meals, this sandwich really satisfies. You can pair the chickpea salad with wheat crackers or cucumber slices for a great snack. I also love it stuffed in a pita pocket or layered on crusty bread with tons of crisp veggies and sliced dill pickles—my sandwich essential.

CHICKPEA SALAD:

1 (15-ounce) can chickpeas, drained and rinsed

¼ cup plain whole-milk or 2% Greek yogurt

2 tablespoons mayonnaise

1 teaspoon whole-grain mustard

2 tablespoons finely chopped dill

1 tablespoon finely chopped parsley

1 celery stalk, diced

1 small shallot, minced

Salt and black pepper

SANDWICHES:

6 or 8 slices bread, toasted

Sliced tomatoes

Pickles

Sliced red onion

Sprouts

Sliced avocado

1. In a large bowl, mix together the chickpeas, yogurt, mayonnaise, mustard, dill, and parsley. Using a potato masher or the back of a fork, mash the chickpeas until chunky and well combined with the other ingredients. Stir in the celery and shallot and season with salt and pepper to taste.

2. Take a slice of bread and spread a scoop of the chickpea salad evenly on it. Top the salad with the tomato slices, pickles, red onion slices, sprouts, and avocado slices; cap off with another slice of bread. Repeat with the remaining ingredients to make 3 or 4 sandwiches.

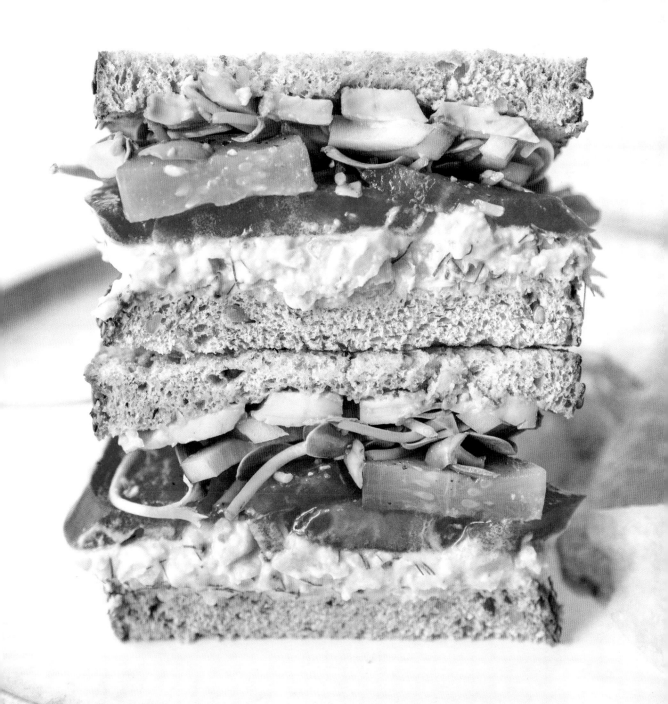

Soy-Ginger Tuna Burgers
WITH SRIRACHA MAYO

MAKES 4 burgers   PREP TIME: 30 minutes   COOK TIME: 10 minutes

Thank God for canned tuna. Used to make a basic tuna salad, added to mac and cheese, or served as part of my favorite easy-yet-fancy, tapas-inspired dinner of olive oil–packed tuna and roasted tomatoes over crusty bread, canned tuna has worked hard over the years to keep me fed! In writing this book, I knew I wanted to perfect a burger made with canned tuna, and I finally got it with this recipe. With fresh herbs, soy, and ginger, these tuna burgers are super flavorful; thanks to the egg and panko binder, they're also moist and juicy.

Feel free to use any type of canned tuna you like. If using solid white tuna, drain it well and shred the fish steak with a fork into small flakes. If using chunk light tuna, which is already flaky, drain it very well, pressing down on the fish with the back of a spoon to get out as much liquid as you can. When the tuna flakes are well drained, they stick together well, which makes it easier to form the patties (if you still have a hard time forming the patties, add a bit of mayo to help bind the fish flakes). To dress up this recipe further, a slice of grilled pineapple would be an epic addition. You could also layer some sweet potato chips over the avocado to add some crunch.

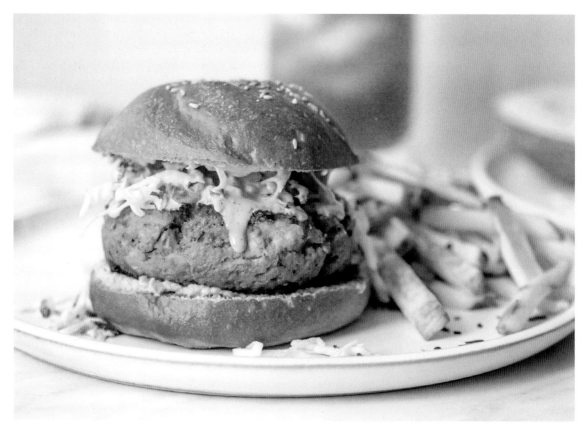

CILANTRO-LIME SLAW:

2 cups shredded cabbage

1 scallion, thinly sliced

2 tablespoons chopped cilantro

Juice of ½ lime

1 teaspoon toasted sesame oil

Salt

BURGER PATTIES:

4 (5-ounce) cans tuna in water, drained well

2 scallions, thinly sliced

2 tablespoons chopped cilantro

2 tablespoons soy sauce

2 tablespoons grated ginger

2 cloves garlic, minced

½ cup panko breadcrumbs

3 large eggs, lightly beaten

2 tablespoons neutral-flavored oil, like canola or avocado oil

1 avocado, halved, pitted, and peeled

4 burger buns, toasted

SRIRACHA MAYO:

¼ cup mayonnaise

2 tablespoons Sriracha sauce

1. Make the slaw: In a medium bowl, combine the cabbage, scallion, and cilantro. Add the lime juice, sesame oil, and a large pinch of salt and toss to combine. Set aside to let the slaw marinate.

2. Make the burger patties: In a large bowl, mix together the tuna, scallions, cilantro, soy sauce, ginger, and garlic with a fork. Mix in the panko and eggs until well combined and the tuna sticks together. Divide into 4 even portions, roll each into a ball, and set aside.

3. Heat the oil in a large skillet over medium-high heat. When the oil is hot, add the tuna balls and press down with the back of a spatula to form 2-inch-thick patties. Cook until the exteriors are golden brown and crispy, 4 to 5 minutes per side.

4. While the burgers are cooking, whisk together the mayonnaise and Sriracha and set aside.

5. To assemble the burgers, mash a quarter of the avocado onto each of the bottom buns and top with a tuna patty. Layer about a quarter of the slaw on top of each patty. Drizzle a quarter of the Sriracha mayo over the slaw and finish with the bun tops.

White Pizza with
FENNEL-ARUGULA SALAD

MAKES one 12-inch pizza (2 to 4 servings) PREP TIME: 15 minutes COOK TIME: 12 minutes

I was turned on to the concept of a pizza salad by my favorite local pizza joint, where they offer the option of ordering one of their New York–style pizzas with a scoop of chopped salad on top. Salad with a pizza is a nice way to incorporate produce into your meal; salad on a pizza is a gourmet topping. My favorite salad for topping pizza is this classic mix of fennel and arugula. The fennel adds crunch, while the arugula adds a peppery flavor. The balsamic dressing melts into the lemony ricotta and mozzarella, flavoring each bite. Remember, vegetables should add to your enjoyment of a meal rather than being an afterthought.

BALSAMIC VINAIGRETTE:

¼ cup extra-virgin olive oil

2 tablespoons balsamic vinegar, plus extra for drizzling

½ teaspoon Dijon mustard

½ teaspoon honey

Salt and black pepper

1 (16-ounce) ball pizza dough, at room temperature

All-purpose flour, for rolling the dough

Cornmeal, for dusting

1 to 2 teaspoons extra-virgin olive oil

1 cup ricotta cheese

2 cloves garlic, minced

Grated zest of 1 lemon

⅛ teaspoon red pepper flakes

8 ounces shredded mozzarella cheese

3 cups lightly packed arugula

1 cup thinly sliced fennel bulb

1. Position an oven rack in the middle of the oven. Preheat the oven to 450°F.

2. Make the vinaigrette: Put the olive oil, vinegar, mustard, and honey in a small jar and shake until well combined. Season with salt and pepper to taste.

3. Dust the pizza dough with a bit of flour. Form it into a smooth ball, then roll into a 12-inch disc on a pizza stone dusted with cornmeal to prevent sticking. (If you don't have a pizza stone, use a large heavy-gauge baking sheet lined with parchment paper.) Drizzle the olive oil over the dough and spread the oil evenly with your fingers.

4. In a bowl, mix the ricotta, garlic, lemon zest, and red pepper flakes until well combined. Spread the mixture evenly over the dough, leaving a ½- to ¾-inch border. Sprinkle the mozzarella evenly over the ricotta mixture.

5. Bake the pizza until the crust is golden and the cheese melted and bubbly, 10 to 12 minutes.

6. When the pizza is almost done, toss the arugula and fennel with the vinaigrette.

7. Remove the pizza from the oven and immediately transfer it to a serving platter. While the pizza is still hot, top it with the salad. Give it a light drizzle of balsamic vinegar and serve immediately.

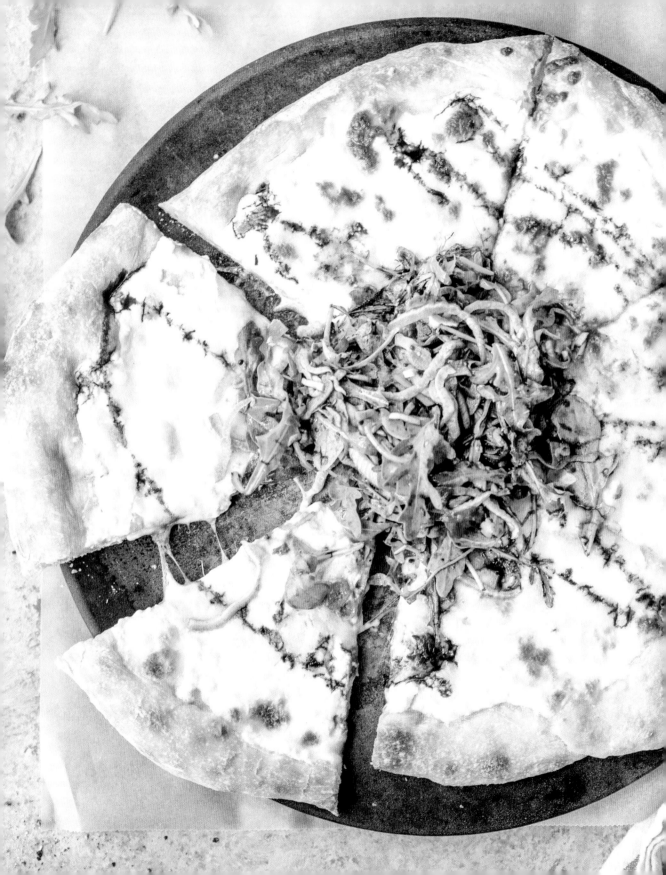

Three Easy
PASTA SAUCES

Sure, you can use pasta sauce from the jar; that is 1,000 percent acceptable. In fact, many store-bought sauces are incredibly tasty. But there's something special about making your own sauce from scratch. And when you do, make things easy on yourself and keep the rest of the dish simple. Just add freshly cooked pasta, roasted vegetables, and your protein of choice. The following recipes are for three of my favorite pasta sauces—the ones I keep coming back to again and again.

For gentle nutrition, I generally like to encourage whole grains. However, when considering whether or not to use whole-grain pasta, think about flavor first, then determine whether it will complement your dish. When it comes to pasta and sauce pairings, I've found that whole-grain pasta has a nutty flavor that can overwhelm some delicate sauces. It prefers more rustic sauces, like the kale and hazelnut pesto or the tomato-basil sauce I've included here, especially with the addition of braised beef or browned ground beef. Creamy sauces, like the Parmesan pepper cream sauce, on the other hand, would be totally overwhelmed by the whole-grain flavor; it pairs better with regular white-flour pasta.

Parmesan Pepper Cream Sauce

MAKES about 2⅓ cups   PREP TIME: 10 minutes   COOK TIME: 5 minutes

This sauce is sort of a mix of cacio e pepe, the classic Italian dish of spaghetti tossed with butter, Parmesan, and pepper, and Alfredo sauce. To make pasta with this cream sauce even more delicious and hearty, you can add some crispy roasted broccoli and top it off with sliced roasted chicken breast.

2 tablespoons extra-virgin olive oil

1 clove garlic, minced

2 tablespoons all-purpose flour

2 cups whole or 2% milk

1 cup grated Parmesan cheese

1 teaspoon ground black pepper, or more to taste

Salt

1. Heat the olive oil in a medium skillet over medium-high heat. Add the garlic and cook for 30 seconds, until fragrant. Whisk in the flour and cook, whisking constantly, for 1 minute.

2. Whisk in the milk and bring to a boil. Reduce the heat and simmer until slightly thickened, about 2 minutes. Whisk in the Parmesan cheese and pepper until the cheese melts, about 30 seconds. Taste and season with salt. Toss with pasta and serve immediately.

Kale-Hazelnut Pesto

MAKES 1⅓ cups   PREP TIME: 15 minutes

When I make pesto, it's often to use up extra greens or herbs that are about to go bad. I rarely follow a recipe; I just blend greens with toasted nuts, minced garlic, Parmesan, and olive oil—plus a little lemon juice for a hit of acid and to keep the sauce bright green in the fridge. This combination of kale and hazelnut is one I always come back to. Pasta with kale-hazelnut pesto is delicious served simply— or perhaps with some extra hazelnuts on top. If you want to kick it up, throw in some roasted cherry tomatoes and mini fresh mozzarella balls.

2 cloves garlic, minced

⅓ cup toasted hazelnuts

½ cup grated Parmesan cheese

5 cups roughly chopped kale leaves

½ teaspoon salt

¼ teaspoon ground black pepper

Juice of ½ lemon

⅓ cup extra-virgin olive oil

Place the garlic, hazelnuts, Parmesan, kale, salt, and pepper in a food processor; pulse until roughly chopped. Add the lemon juice and blend, then add the olive oil in a thin stream until the pesto is creamy, stopping to scrape down the sides as needed.

The Best Tomato Basil Sauce

MAKES about 3½ cups   PREP TIME: 15 minutes   COOK TIME: 30 minutes

Want to know how to make the most delicious tomato basil sauce? Just add butter! Working in tandem with olive oil, butter cuts the acidic bite of the tomatoes and elevates the sauce by creating a luxurious texture and rich flavor. The other trick is to use San Marzano tomatoes. If you've ever noticed them at the store, you may have wondered if they're really worth three times the price of your grocery store brand. Yes, yes, they are, especially in a dish where tomatoes are the star. San Marzanos have a richer, sweeter, more, well, tomatoey flavor. I suggest doubling the recipe and freezing the extra sauce.

2 tablespoons extra-virgin olive oil

2 tablespoons unsalted butter

½ large yellow onion, finely chopped

1¼ teaspoons salt, divided

5 cloves garlic, minced

¼ teaspoon red pepper flakes

2 (28-ounce) cans whole peeled San Marzano tomatoes

¼ cup loosely packed basil leaves, roughly chopped

1 teaspoon granulated sugar

¼ teaspoon ground black pepper

1. Heat the olive oil and butter in a medium pot over medium-high heat. When the butter melts and is sizzling, add the onion and ¼ teaspoon of the salt and sauté until translucent, about 5 minutes. Stir in the garlic and red pepper flakes and cook until fragrant, about 1 minute.

2. Stir in the tomatoes, basil, sugar, the remaining 1 teaspoon of salt, and the pepper. Break up the tomatoes slightly with the back of a wooden spoon. Bring to a simmer, reduce the heat to medium, and cook until thickened slightly and the flavors have melded together, 20 to 25 minutes.

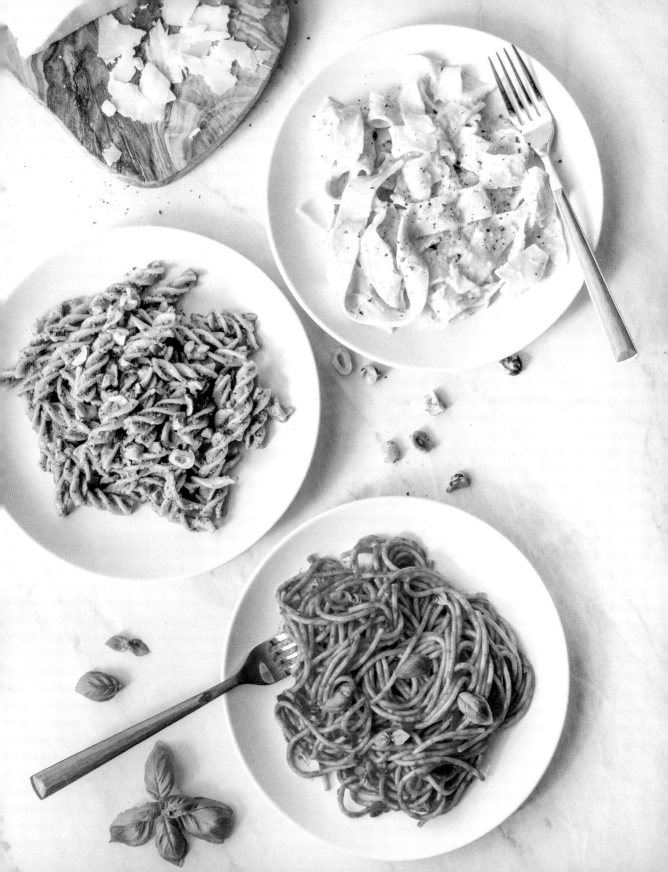

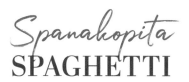

Spanakopita SPAGHETTI

MAKES 3 to 4 servings PREP TIME: 15 minutes COOK TIME: 15 minutes

Spaghetti with canned white beans and sautéed frozen spinach flavored with garlic and onions has been a go-to dinner for me since college. I wanted to share an upgraded spin on it in this book, considering it's a recipe that's fed me on many, many busy nights. Inspired by spanakopita, the classic Greek spinach pastry, I came up with this dish. I thought it was pretty incredible, but now that one of my recipe testers has told me that the flavors are spot on for the spanakopita recipe that has been passed down through the generations in her family, I am feeling absolutely cocky about this recipe!

8 ounces whole-grain spaghetti

¼ cup extra-virgin olive oil

½ large yellow onion, diced

Salt

4 cloves garlic, thinly sliced

1 (6-ounce) bag frozen baby spinach, thawed and squeezed dry

2 scallions, chopped

¼ cup chopped dill

¼ cup chopped parsley

2 tablespoons chopped mint

1 (15-ounce) can cannellini beans, drained and rinsed

Juice of ½ lemon

Black pepper

½ cup crumbled feta cheese

⅓ cup toasted walnuts, chopped

1.   Cook the spaghetti according to the package instructions until al dente. Reserve ½ cup of the starchy pasta water, drain the pasta, and set aside.

2.   While the pasta is cooking, heat the olive oil in a large skillet over medium-high heat. Add the onion, along with a pinch of salt, and cook until translucent, about 5 minutes. Add the garlic and continue cooking until the onion is lightly golden, 3 to 5 minutes longer. Add the spinach, scallions, and herbs; cook, stirring occasionally, until wilted, about 5 minutes. Stir in the beans and cook until warmed through, about 1 minute.

3.   Stir in the spaghetti along with the lemon juice and just enough of the reserved pasta water to make the mixture saucy enough to cling to the pasta. Season with salt and pepper to taste. Divide the spaghetti among 3 or 4 bowls and serve topped with the feta and walnuts.

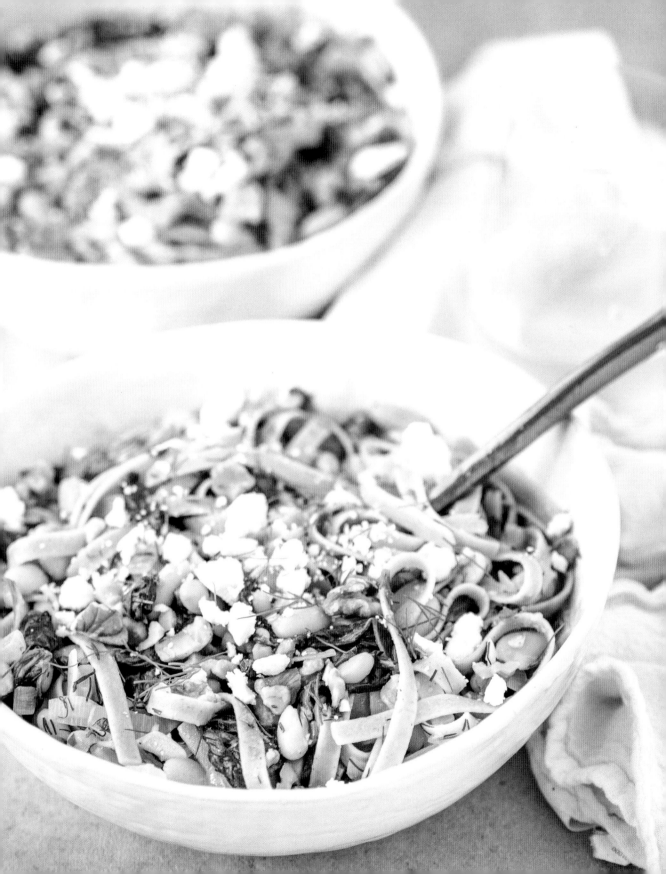

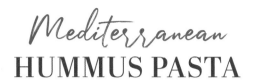

Mediterranean
HUMMUS PASTA

MAKES 3 to 4 servings   PREP TIME: 15 minutes   COOK TIME: 10 minutes

Continuing the theme of quick and easy pasta recipes is this Mediterranean hummus pasta. I used to make a pasta recipe that called for a hummus-inspired chickpea sauce almost every other week. One day, I had extra hummus in my fridge and had the inspired thought to use that instead! It was a total time-saver, and the sauce made from store-bought hummus was just as creamy, luxurious, garlicky, and delicious on pasta.

I use this recipe as a template, switching up the sautéed vegetables and hummus flavors to keep things interesting. Try sautéed asparagus with lemony hummus and goat cheese or spicy red pepper hummus with roasted eggplant.

8 ounces whole-grain penne pasta

1 tablespoon extra-virgin olive oil

1 large zucchini, cubed

1 cup cherry tomatoes, halved

¼ cup sliced Kalamata olives

½ cup roasted garlic hummus

Chopped parsley, cilantro, and/ or mint, for garnish (optional)

1. Cook the pasta according to the package instructions until al dente. Reserve ½ cup of the starchy cooking water, drain the pasta, and set aside.

2. While the pasta is cooking, heat the olive oil in a large skillet over medium-high heat. Add the zucchini and tomatoes and sauté until the zucchini is golden brown and tender, 5 to 7 minutes. Stir in the olives and turn off the heat.

3. Add the drained pasta to the cooked vegetables. Stir in the hummus and just enough of the reserved pasta water to make the mixture just saucy enough to cling to the pasta. Turn the heat to medium-low and cook until warmed through, about 1 minute. Serve garnished with the fresh herbs, if desired.

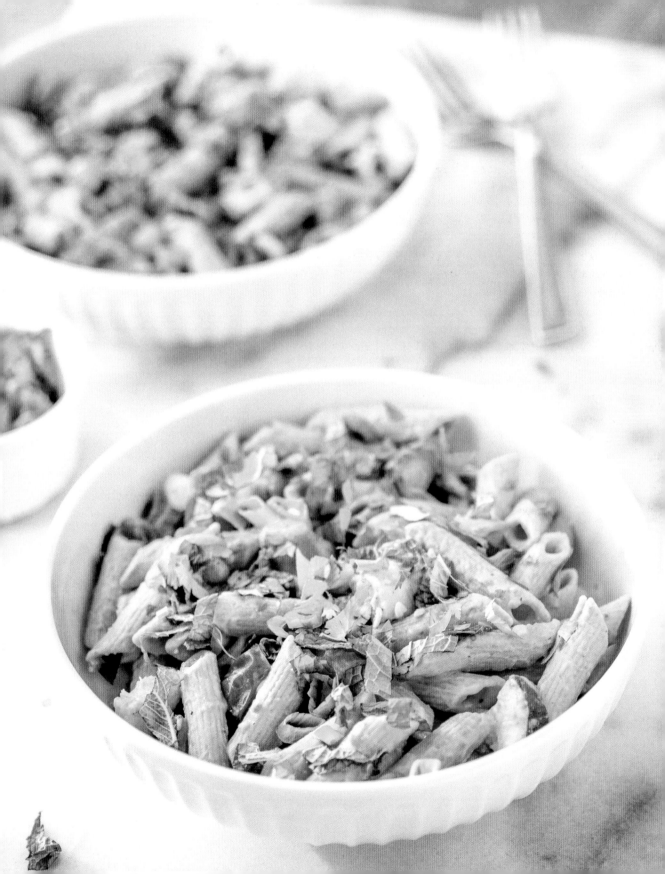

Pumpkin Gnocchi with
BRUSSELS SPROUTS & SAUSAGE

MAKES 3 to 4 servings PREP TIME: 20 minutes COOK TIME: 30 minutes

Gnocchi is my all-time favorite pasta. In this recipe, it is combined with a creamy pumpkin sauce, salty and savory sweet Italian sausage, and slightly bitter roasted Brussels sprouts into pure comfort in a bowl. For a vegetarian version, feel free to use vegan sausage. However, don't be afraid to enjoy regular sausage in this dish. Although processed meats get bad press, remember that they're just one type of protein among the many you're eating. Focus on eating a variety of proteins, and sausage can be one of them!

This recipe makes more pumpkin sauce than you'll need. It freezes beautifully for future pasta making.

½ pound Brussels sprouts, trimmed and quartered (keep a little of the stem intact to hold the quarters together)

3 tablespoons extra-virgin olive oil, divided

Salt and black pepper

1 (1-pound) package dried gnocchi

8 ounces precooked sweet Italian sausage links, sliced into ½-inch rounds

½ large sweet onion, finely diced

6 cloves garlic, thinly sliced

1 tablespoon chopped sage

1 (15-ounce) can pumpkin puree (not pumpkin pie filling)

1 cup low-sodium chicken or vegetable broth

1 jarred roasted red pepper, drained and finely diced

¼ cup heavy cream or mascarpone

Grated or shaved Parmesan cheese, for serving

1. Preheat the oven to 400°F.

2. Toss the Brussels sprouts with 1 tablespoon of the olive oil and season with salt and pepper. Spread evenly on a sheet pan and roast, flipping halfway through the cooking time, until tender and golden, 15 to 20 minutes.

3. Bring a large pot of salted water to a boil.

4. While the Brussels sprouts are roasting and the water is coming to a boil, heat 1 tablespoon of the olive oil in a medium saucepan over medium-high heat. Add the sausage and cook, stirring occasionally, until browned and heated through, 5 to 7 minutes. Remove from the pan and set aside. Wipe the pan clean with paper towel.

5. In the same pan, heat the remaining 1 tablespoon of olive oil over medium-high heat. Add the onion along with a pinch of salt and cook until the onion is translucent, 4 to 5 minutes. Stir in the garlic and sage and cook for 1 minute more.

6. Scrape the contents of the pan into a blender or food processor. Add the pumpkin puree, broth, red pepper, and cream and blend until smooth. Season with salt and pepper to taste.

7. When the water reaches a boil, add the gnocchi and cook according to the package instructions. Drain and return to the pot. Stir in the roasted Brussels sprouts, sausage, and enough of the pumpkin sauce to make it creamy. Warm through over medium heat. Serve sprinkled with Parmesan cheese.

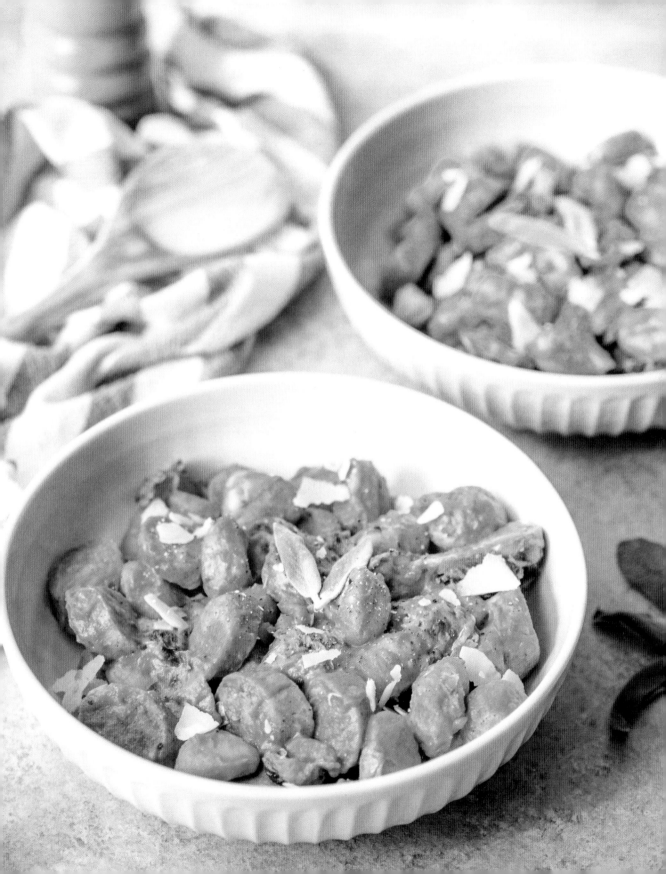

Gingery Fried Rice with
CAULIFLOWER RICE

MAKES 3 to 4 servings   PREP TIME: 30 minutes   COOK TIME: 15 minutes

I promise I'm not about to espouse the benefits of swapping rice with cauliflower rice. However, I am going to espouse the benefits of enjoying cauliflower rice with your regular rice. This recipe uses a mixture of riced cauliflower and cooked white or brown rice as a way to work some veggies into an easy weeknight meal. I'm a bit embarrassed to admit this as a loud and proud non-diet dietitian, but I really do enjoy cauliflower rice. The little cauliflower bits take on tons of flavor when fried with garlic and onions. It's also an incredibly convenient vegetable to have on hand. A bag of riced cauliflower keeps well in the fridge, and frozen riced cauliflower tastes just as good as fresh. That said, as tasty and convenient as cauliflower rice is, your body still needs carbs. So let's not use cauliflower as a rice swap unless you're adding something else with carbs to your plate. There may be foods associated with dieting that you legitimately enjoy. Intuitive eating doesn't make those foods off-limits; it just asks you to question your motives in choosing them.

Be sure to use cold cooked rice or frozen rice in this recipe. Hot, freshly cooked rice won't crisp up, and your fried rice will have a sticky, pasty texture.

3 tablespoons toasted sesame oil, divided

1 pound fresh or frozen riced cauliflower

2 carrots, halved lengthwise and thinly sliced

Salt

⅓ cup thinly sliced scallions, plus extra for serving if desired

3 tablespoons grated ginger

3 cloves garlic, minced

3 cups cold cooked white or brown rice

1 cup frozen edamame, thawed

1 cup frozen peas, thawed

3 to 4 tablespoons soy sauce

Black pepper

3 large eggs, beaten and seasoned with salt and black pepper

Sriracha sauce, for serving (optional)

Toasted sesame seeds, for garnish (optional)

1. Heat 1 tablespoon of the sesame oil in a large nonstick skillet over medium-high heat. Add the riced cauliflower and carrots along with a pinch of salt and cook, stirring occasionally, until the cauliflower is lightly golden, about 5 minutes. Stir in the scallions, ginger, and garlic and cook, stirring occasionally, until fragrant, about 2 minutes. Scrape into a large serving bowl and set aside.

2. Wipe the skillet clean with a paper towel, add 1 tablespoon of the sesame oil, and warm over medium-high heat. Add the rice and a pinch of salt and cook, stirring occasionally, until lightly golden and crispy, about 5 minutes. Stir in the edamame and peas and cook for an additional 2 minutes to warm through. Stir in the soy sauce. Taste and season with additional salt and pepper as needed. Scrape the fried rice into the same serving bowl and set aside.

3. Wipe the skillet clean and add the remaining 1 tablespoon of sesame oil. Warm over medium-high heat and pour in the beaten eggs. Scramble for about a minute, then stir the eggs into the rice. Serve garnished with Sriracha, additional scallions, and toasted sesame seeds, if using.

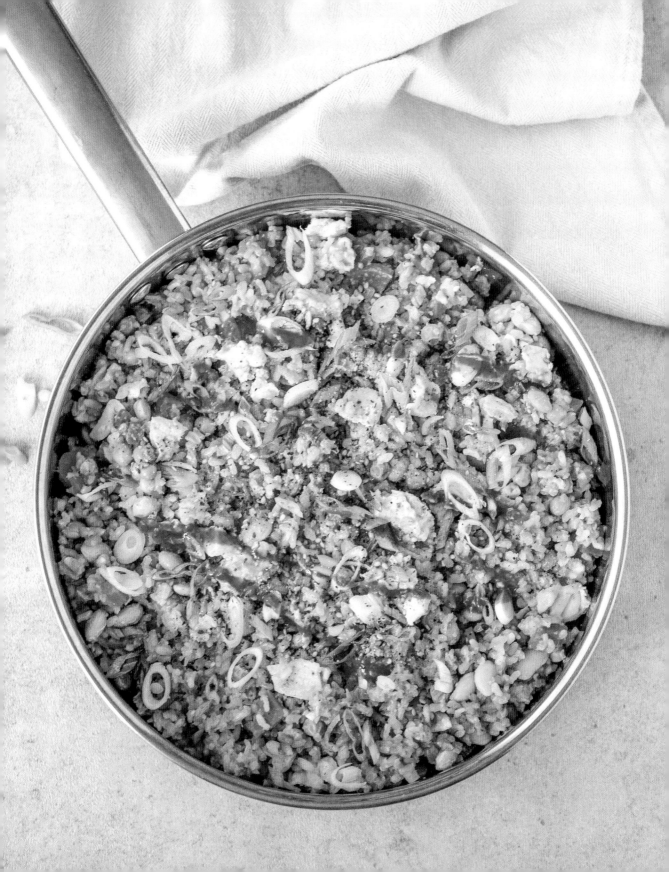

Vegetarian
STUFFED POBLANOS

MAKES 4 stuffed poblanos   PREP TIME: 20 minutes   COOK TIME: 40 minutes

These vegetarian stuffed poblanos are a great example of how processed ingredients can be used to save time in making a nutritious and satisfying dinner. This recipe uses canned refried beans, microwave-in-a-bag rice, and store-bought enchilada sauce. There's a lot of fearmongering around processed ingredients, but, as this recipe shows, they can help you get a tasty home-cooked meal on the table without a lot of hassle.

The only part of this recipe that you may find challenging is peeling the skins off the poblanos. Poblano skins get a little papery when roasted and are unpleasant to eat, so it's best to take the time to remove them. To do so, char the poblanos under the broiler until the skins are blackened, then steam them in a bowl capped with a plate or sealed with plastic wrap. This loosens the skins so they're easy to peel off. I find it super meditative. Maybe you will too!

4 large poblano peppers

1 tablespoon neutral-flavored oil, like canola or avocado oil

½ large yellow onion, diced

1 clove garlic, minced

½ teaspoon chili powder

½ teaspoon ground cumin

1 (16-ounce) can refried black beans

1 (8.8-ounce) microwave-in-the-bag steamed brown or white rice, or 2 cups cooked brown or white rice

Salt and black pepper

1 (13-ounce) bottle enchilada sauce

1 cup shredded sharp cheddar cheese

FOR GARNISH (OPTIONAL):

Chopped cilantro

Thinly sliced scallions

1.   Preheat the broiler. Arrange the poblanos on a sheet pan and place in the oven directly under the broiler until the skins are blackened and charred, about 3 minutes per side. Remove the poblanos from the oven and turn off the broiler.

2.   Place the poblanos in a bowl and cover tightly with a plate or plastic wrap. Leave the peppers to steam for about 10 minutes.

3.   Meanwhile, prepare the filling: Heat the oil in a medium saucepan over medium-high heat. Add the onion and garlic and sauté until lightly golden, about 5 minutes. Stir in the chili powder and cumin and cook until fragrant, about 30 seconds. Stir in the beans and rice, mashing with the back of a spatula or spoon until well combined. Season with salt and pepper to taste.

4.   Preheat the oven to 350°F.

5.   Carefully peel the thin layer of skin off the poblanos (it's okay if you can't get all of it off). Cut a slit in each pepper from the stem all the way to the tip. Using a paring knife, carefully cut away the thick piece of flesh under the stem that's attached to the seeds. Briefly rinse under water to remove any remaining seeds.

6.   Arrange the poblanos in a 7 by 11-inch baking dish. Stuff the bean and rice mixture evenly into the poblanos, patting it in using your hands. Pour the enchilada sauce over and around the stuffed poblanos and top with the cheese. Bake until the sauce is bubbly and the cheese melts and turns lightly golden, about 30 minutes. Serve garnished with the cilantro and scallions, if desired.

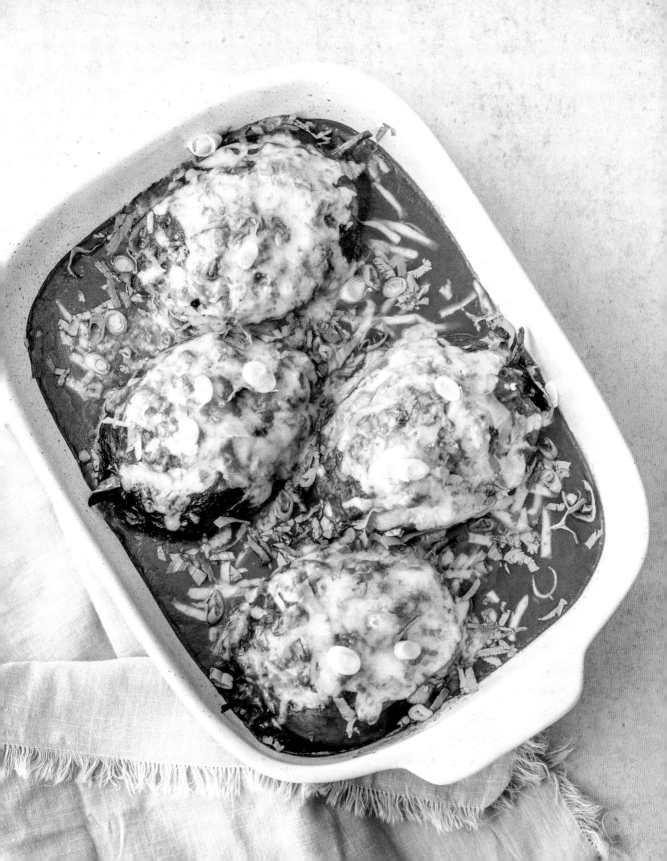

Chickpea & Butternut Squash
MASALA

MAKES 4 to 6 servings   PREP TIME: 20 minutes   COOK TIME: 50 minutes

Carbohydrates are essential for a satisfying meal that keeps your body adequately fueled until the next time you eat. Not only should you not feel guilty for including a carbohydrate in your meal, but you shouldn't feel guilty for having multiple carbs! This chickpea and butternut squash masala contains not one or two, but three carbohydrate sources—four if you serve it with roti or naan, which I highly recommend. Remember that meals naturally vary in macronutrient content, and there's no right or wrong amount. Most healthy eating guidelines, like the US government's MyPlate, teach pairing protein with a single carbohydrate and a vegetable side. But this is a very Eurocentric view, as it is normal in other cultures to eat multiple carbohydrate sources at meals. Think beans and rice in Latin America; lentil stews served with injera, a sourdough flatbread made from teff; and, of course, Indian curries made with lentils, beans, or potatoes, often served over rice or with flatbread.

Feel free to add different proteins and vegetables to this masala. Try chicken, tofu, paneer cheese, or lamb meatballs to switch it up. For vegetables, this recipe is also tasty made with spinach, carrots, peas, or zucchini. You might want to make extra sauce to freeze for later use.

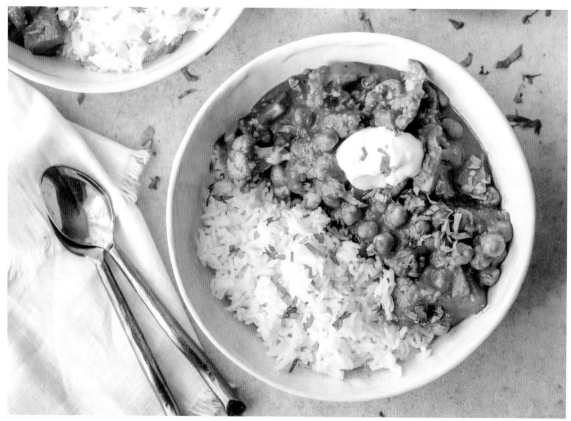

2 tablespoons neutral-flavored oil, like canola or avocado oil, or ghee

½ large yellow onion, chopped

¼ cup minced ginger

6 cloves garlic, minced

½ teaspoon plus 1 pinch of salt, divided

1 teaspoon garam masala

1 teaspoon ground cumin

1 teaspoon paprika

½ teaspoon ground cinnamon

⅛ to ¼ teaspoon cayenne pepper, depending on heat preference

1 (15-ounce) can crushed tomatoes

½ cup water

1 (13.5-ounce) can full-fat coconut milk

¼ teaspoon ground black pepper

1 small butternut squash, peeled, deseeded, and cut into ¾-inch cubes

1 head cauliflower, trimmed, cored, and cut into florets roughly the same size as the squash

1 (15-ounce) can chickpeas, drained and rinsed

FOR GARNISH/SERVING:

Cooked basmati rice

Chopped cilantro (optional)

Plain whole-milk or 2% Greek yogurt (optional)

Naan, roti, or other Indian bread (optional)

1. Heat the oil in a 4-quart Dutch oven or large saucepan over medium-high heat. Add the onion, ginger, garlic, and a pinch of salt. Cook, stirring occasionally, until golden brown, about 10 minutes. Stir in the spices and cook until fragrant, about 1 minute.

2. Add the crushed tomatoes and water, scraping up any browned bits at the bottom of the pan. Bring to a boil, reduce the heat, and simmer to thicken, about 10 minutes.

3. Carefully transfer the tomato sauce to a blender. Add the coconut milk, the remaining ½ teaspoon of salt, and the pepper; blend until smooth.

4. Pour the sauce back into the pan. Return to a boil and stir in the butternut squash and cauliflower. Reduce the heat, partially cover, and simmer until tender, about 25 minutes.

5. Stir in the chickpeas and cook for 5 minutes to warm through. Season with more salt and pepper to taste. Serve over rice and garnish with cilantro and yogurt, if using. Serve with Indian bread on the side, if desired.

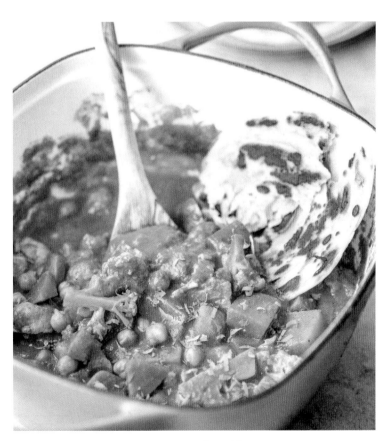

Goat Cheese Grits with
SPRING VEGETABLES &
ROASTED RED PEPPER SAUCE

MAKES 3 to 4 servings, plus extra sauce   PREP TIME: 45 minutes   COOK TIME: 30 minutes

To include more whole grains in your meals, look beyond whole-grain bread, brown rice, and whole-wheat pasta. There's a world of whole grains out there! Living in South Carolina, I had to use this book as an opportunity to highlight grits. They're a bit of a religion where I live. In fact, our downtown skyline in Columbia (if you want to call it that) is capped off by an old grits mill. If you've tried only instant grits, you're missing out. Stone-ground grits are much creamier and more flavorful, and they're a whole grain! Made from ground corn (i.e., cornmeal), stone-ground grits contain all parts of the grain, so they're packed with nutrients.

This recipe, featuring the bright flavors and colors of spring produce, was inspired by the goat cheese grits bowl served at one of my favorite restaurants in Asheville, North Carolina: Tupelo Honey.

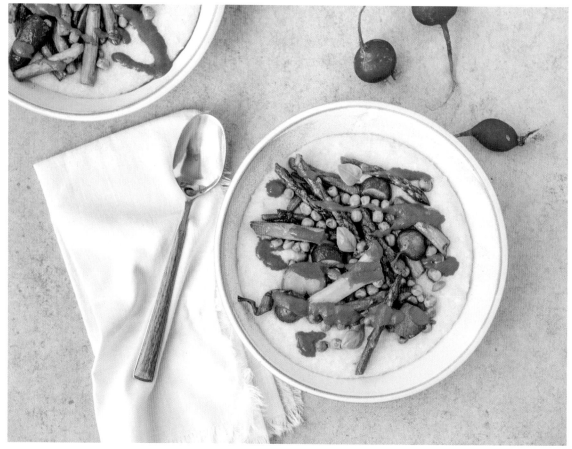

GRITS:

2 cups whole or 2% milk

2 cups water

¼ teaspoon salt

1 cup stone-ground grits

⅓ cup crumbled goat cheese

Salt and black pepper

ROASTED RED PEPPER SAUCE:

1 (12-ounce) jar roasted red peppers, drained

¼ cup packed basil leaves, plus extra for garnish

2 tablespoons extra-virgin olive oil

1 clove garlic, minced

¼ teaspoon salt

SPRING VEGETABLES:

1 tablespoon unsalted butter

1 tablespoon extra-virgin olive oil

1 bundle asparagus, woody stems snapped off, cut into 1-inch pieces

8 ounces radishes, halved (or quartered if large)

3 scallions, cut into 1-inch pieces

¾ cup frozen peas

⅓ cup low-sodium vegetable or chicken broth

Salt and black pepper

1.   Make the grits: Bring the milk, water, and salt to a boil in a medium pot over medium-high heat. Add the grits in a thin stream, whisking constantly; reduce the heat to medium and cook, stirring every couple of minutes, until thick and creamy, 25 to 30 minutes. Stir in the goat cheese and season with more salt and pepper to taste.

2.   While the grits are cooking, prepare the sauce: Put the roasted red peppers, basil leaves, olive oil, garlic, and salt in a blender and blend until smooth. Set aside.

3.   Prepare the vegetables: Heat the butter and olive oil in a large nonstick skillet over medium-high heat until the butter melts and sizzles. Add the asparagus and radishes and sauté until lightly golden, 4 to 5 minutes. Stir in the scallions, peas, and broth. Cook, stirring occasionally, until the liquid has mostly evaporated and the vegetables are crisp-tender, 4 to 5 minutes, adding more broth as needed to prevent them from drying out. Season with salt and pepper to taste.

4.   Divide the grits among 3 or 4 bowls. Top with the sautéed vegetables. Drizzle with some of the roasted red pepper sauce. (You will have some sauce left over; store it in a lidded container in the fridge for up to a week, or freeze for a few months.) Garnish with the basil and serve.

Lentil & Mushroom
RAGU–STUFFED POTATOES

MAKES 4 stuffed potatoes   PREP TIME: 30 minutes   COOK TIME: 1 hour 20 minutes

Can you tell from reading this book that I really love stuffed baked potatoes? I think I have mentioned them as a meal idea at least three or four times! While I have been known to stuff canned chili into a potato cooked in the microwave and call it dinner, this recipe for baked potatoes filled with a lentil and mushroom ragu is for when I want to put in a little more effort and get more of a reward.

Quick-cooking lentils are a weeknight-friendly legume. Beyond Indian dal and lentil soup, lentils can be used as a tasty vegetarian substitute for meat in most recipes, like this ragu, which is usually made with ground beef. The ragu gets an additional dose of meaty flavor from cremini mushrooms.

If you prefer sweet potatoes, they also work well in this recipe. However, don't be afraid to enjoy white potatoes, another food that's unfairly maligned! Sweet potatoes get put on a nutritional pedestal even though, other than being packed with vitamin A, they and their white counterparts are essentially equal nutritionally.

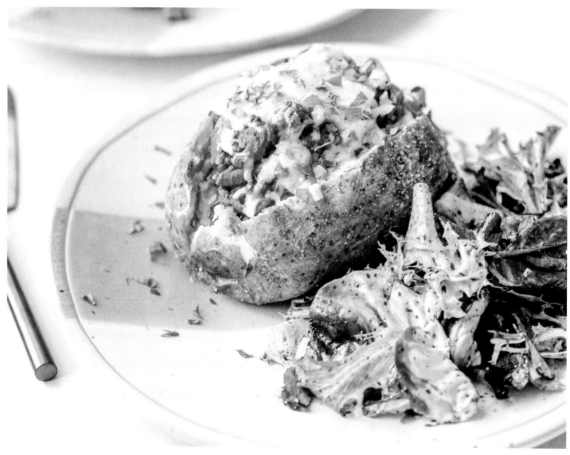

POTATOES:

4 medium russet potatoes

Extra-virgin olive oil

Salt and black pepper

RAGU:

2 tablespoons extra-virgin olive oil

½ large yellow onion, diced

1 medium carrot, diced

4 cloves garlic, minced

½ teaspoon plus 1 pinch of salt, divided

8 ounces cremini mushrooms, diced

1 bay leaf

½ teaspoon dried basil

½ teaspoon dried oregano

1 to 2 pinches red pepper flakes

1 tablespoon tomato paste

⅓ cup dry red wine

1 (28-ounce) can crushed tomatoes

¼ teaspoon black pepper

1 (15-ounce) can lentils, drained and rinsed

1 cup shredded Gruyère cheese

Chopped parsley, for garnish (optional)

1. Place an oven rack in the middle of the oven. Preheat the oven to 350°F.

2. Scrub the potatoes clean, pat them dry, and prick them all over with a fork. Rub with a thin layer of olive oil and sprinkle generously with salt and pepper. Place on a baking sheet and bake until the skins have crisped up and the potatoes feel tender when pressed, 60 to 75 minutes.

3. While the potatoes are baking, prepare the ragu: Heat the olive oil in a medium saucepan over medium-high heat. Add the onion, carrot, garlic, and a pinch of salt and cook, stirring occasionally, until the onion is translucent, 4 to 5 minutes. Stir in the mushrooms and cook, stirring occasionally, until the mushrooms are tender and the onion is golden, about 5 minutes.

4. Stir in the bay leaf, basil, oregano, and red pepper flakes and cook until fragrant, 30 seconds. Stir in the tomato paste and cook for 1 minute. Pour in the wine and cook, stirring constantly to scrape up any browned bits at the bottom of the pan, until the liquid is mostly absorbed, about 1 minute.

5. Stir in the crushed tomatoes, the remaining ½ teaspoon of salt, and the pepper. Bring to a boil, reduce the heat, and simmer until thickened, about 20 minutes. Remove and discard the bay leaf.

6. Make a lengthwise slit in the top of each potato and squeeze it open from both ends. Spoon in the ragu and top each potato with ¼ cup of the cheese. Place back in the oven and bake until the cheese melts, about 5 minutes. Serve garnished with parsley, if desired.

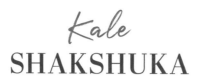

Kale
SHAKSHUKA

———— **MAKES 4 servings   PREP TIME: 15 minutes   COOK TIME: 25 minutes** ————

Shakshuka is a traditional dish of eggs simmered in a spiced tomato sauce that's especially popular in North Africa and the Middle East. It's my favorite way to enjoy breakfast for dinner; there's nothing quite like the taste of runny egg yolks mingling with spicy tomato sauce, briny feta, and fresh herbs—especially when you scoop it all up with warm pita bread. In this recipe, I add kale for a little green and for its slightly bitter flavor that I love in spicy tomato sauces. If you like, you could make and freeze the sauce to use later in future batches of this recipe.

The harissa yogurt in this dish adds both a cooling element and some heat. Harissa is a North African condiment made from roasted red chilies and spices. Different brands vary quite a bit in spiciness, so if you're sensitive, start with a smaller amount and then add more as tolerated. If you can't find harissa, plain Greek yogurt will work just fine. I like to garnish this with za'atar, a Middle Eastern spice blend of toasted sesame seeds, sumac, oregano, and thyme.

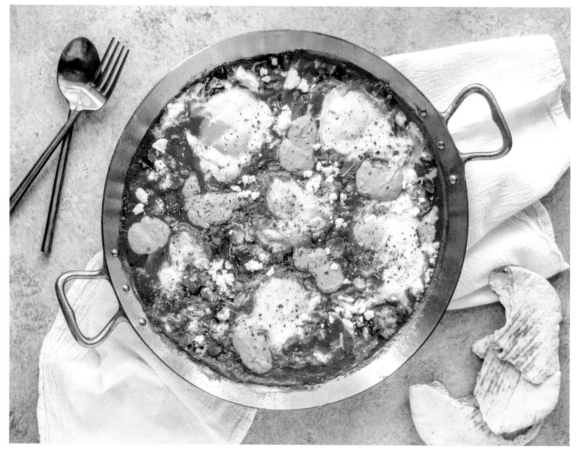

1 tablespoon extra-virgin olive oil

½ large yellow onion, diced

½ red bell pepper, stemmed, deseeded, and diced

1 jalapeño pepper, stemmed, deseeded, and minced

2 cloves garlic, minced

Pinch of salt

1 teaspoon ground cumin

½ teaspoon ground coriander

½ teaspoon smoked paprika

¼ teaspoon red pepper flakes

5 ounces roughly chopped kale, thick stems removed

½ cup low-sodium chicken or vegetable broth

2½ cups tomato basil sauce, store-bought or homemade (page 194)

6 large eggs

¾ cup crumbled feta cheese

HARISSA YOGURT:

½ cup plain whole-milk or 2% Greek yogurt

1½ tablespoons harissa

Pinch of salt

Za'atar, for garnish (optional)

Chopped mint and/or cilantro, for garnish (optional)

Toasted pita bread, for serving

1. Heat the olive oil in a large nonstick skillet over medium-high heat. Add the onion, bell pepper, jalapeño, garlic, and salt. Cook, stirring occasionally, until the onion is translucent, about 5 minutes.

2. Stir in the cumin, coriander, paprika, and red pepper flakes and cook until fragrant, 30 seconds to 1 minute.

3. Stir in the kale and broth. Reduce the heat to medium, cover, and cook until the kale is tender, 7 to 10 minutes, adding more water or broth if it gets too dry.

4. While the kale is cooking, make the harissa yogurt: Whisk together the yogurt and harissa. Season with a pinch of salt.

5. Stir the tomato sauce into the skillet with the kale mixture and bring to a simmer. Make 6 wells for the eggs and crack an egg into each. Sprinkle the feta over the top. Cover and cook until the whites are set and the yolks are slightly runny, 6 to 10 minutes.

6. Put the harissa yogurt on the shakshuka in small dollops. Sprinkle the za'atar and herbs, if using, on top. Serve with the toasted pita.

Slow-Roasted Lemon-Dill
SALMON & SQUASH

———— MAKES 4 servings PREP TIME: 20 minutes, plus 15 minutes to drain squash COOK TIME: 30 minutes ————

Everyone knows the benefits of eating omega-3 rich fatty fish, like salmon, but it's the tough, dried-out salmon that many of us have often encountered that makes the idea of including it in gentle nutrition not so appealing. I love how restaurants are able to get that perfect sear on the fish with crispy skin and juicy flesh, but after years of attempts, I've given up trying to re-create that result in my kitchen. Thankfully, my friend and fellow intuitive eating counselor Kara Lydon taught me a better way to cook salmon at home: slow-roasting.

When salmon is cooked over high heat, the proteins coil up, causing the fish to secrete oil. Slow-roasting cooks the proteins more slowly, which helps the fish retain moisture. It gives the salmon a melt-in-your-mouth texture that's to die for. As a bonus, it doesn't stink up your house the way pan-frying salmon does!

In this recipe, salmon is slow-roasted over a bed of grated squash and white beans flavored simply with herbs, lemon, and garlic. Don't skip the step of squeezing the liquid from the grated squash. Squash has a very high water content, so, without draining and squeezing, you'd end up with a soupy mess. I've suggested a baking time of twenty-five to thirty minutes for medium doneness, but it may take a little bit longer depending on the thickness of your salmon. I like to serve this with jasmine or basmati rice.

---

1 pound mixed zucchini and yellow squash, grated

¼ teaspoon salt

1 (15-ounce) can white beans, drained and rinsed

¼ cup plus 1 tablespoon chopped dill, divided

2 scallions, thinly sliced

1 clove garlic, minced

1 tablespoon extra-virgin olive oil, plus extra for drizzling

1 lemon, halved

¼ teaspoon ground black pepper

4 (6-ounce) skin-on salmon fillets

1. Toss the grated squash with the salt in a large colander and set the colander over a bowl. Let the squash sit for 15 minutes to release some of the liquid.

2. Preheat the oven to 300°F. Pile the squash in the middle of a clean dish towel. Wrap the towel around the squash and squeeze out as much of the liquid as you can. Transfer the squash to a 9 by 13-inch baking dish and fluff it with a fork.

3. Stir the white beans, ¼ cup of the dill, the scallions, garlic, olive oil, the juice of one half of the lemon, and the pepper into the grated squash and spread evenly on the bottom of the baking dish. Nestle the salmon into the squash mixture. Drizzle the salmon with a little bit of olive oil. Sprinkle with salt and pepper, along with the remaining 1 tablespoon of dill. Cut the remaining lemon half into thin slices and place a slice or two on top of each salmon fillet.

4. Bake until the squash is tender and the salmon is slightly opaque and flakes easily with a fork, 25 to 30 minutes.

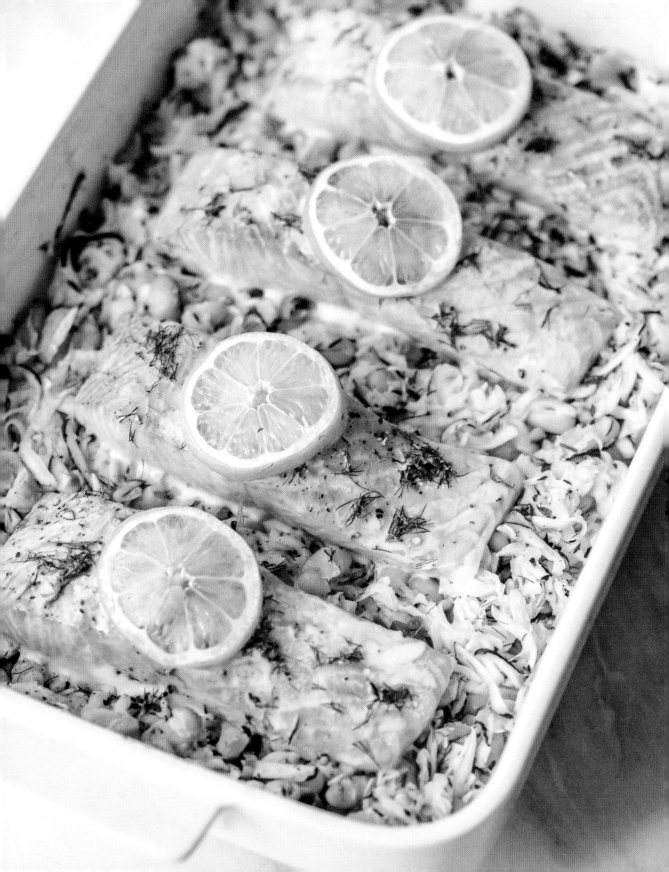

Sheet Pan Maple-Miso Butter Shrimp
WITH GREEN BEANS &
JAPANESE SWEET POTATOES

MAKES 4 servings PREP TIME: 15 minutes COOK TIME: 25 minutes

Miso is one of my essential condiments. Known primarily in the US in the form of miso soup, this Japanese condiment is a paste made from fermented soybeans. If that description isn't selling it to you, I know this recipe for maple-miso butter shrimp will! Miso is salty, nutty, savory, and packed with umami. The maple syrup brings out its natural sweetness and earthiness, while the butter adds richness to the mix. I love to dollop this spread on baked sweet potatoes, baste roasted chicken with it, and add it to roasted Brussels sprouts—it's good tossed with noodles too!

If you can't find Japanese sweet potatoes, regular sweet potatoes will work just fine. However, I highly recommend seeking out the Japanese variety if you can. Japanese sweet potatoes have reddish-purple skin and a creamy-colored flesh that tastes sweeter and nuttier. Many people compare the flavor to that of roasted chestnuts.

1½ pounds Japanese sweet potatoes, halved and sliced into ½-inch-thick half-moons

1 tablespoon neutral-flavored oil, like canola or avocado oil

Salt and black pepper

1½ pounds large shrimp, peeled

12 ounces haricots verts (French green beans), trimmed

Sliced scallions, for garnish

MAPLE-MISO BUTTER:

3 tablespoons miso paste

3 tablespoons unsalted butter

1 tablespoon pure maple syrup

Pinch of red pepper flakes

1. Preheat the oven to 400°F.

2. Toss the sweet potatoes with the oil and season with salt and pepper. Spread evenly on a sheet pan and roast until mostly tender when pierced with a knife and lightly golden, 15 to 20 minutes.

3. While the potatoes are roasting, prepare the maple-miso butter: Put the miso paste, butter, maple syrup, and red pepper flakes in a small saucepan over medium heat. Whisk constantly until the butter melts and the ingredients are well combined; remove from the heat.

4. Put the shrimp and green beans in a large bowl. Add the maple-miso butter and toss to combine.

5. Push the potatoes to one side of the pan. Spread the green beans and shrimp evenly on the other side. Move the oven rack to the top rung and turn on the broiler. Place the pan on the prepared rack and broil until the shrimp are cooked and the green beans are lightly blistered and crisp-tender, about 5 minutes. Garnish with the scallions and serve immediately.

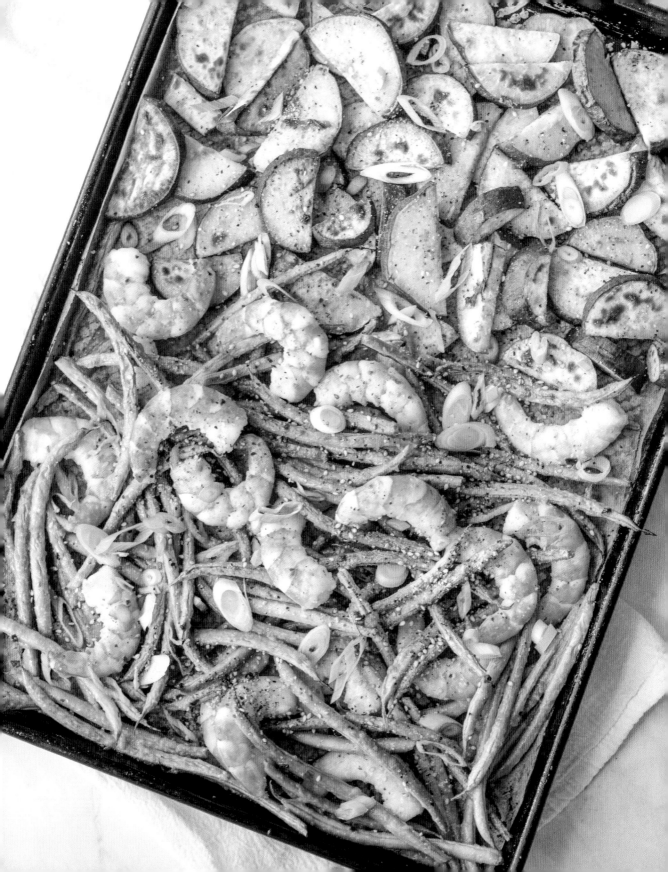

Blackened Fish Tacos
WITH MANGO SALSA

MAKES 8 tacos   PREP TIME: 30 minutes   COOK TIME: 6 minutes

These blackened fish tacos call for a day at the beach and a margarita! While the beach might be harder to come by, hopefully the margarita (virgin or not) is more accessible. Store-bought blackening seasoning makes these tacos easy to throw together in under ten minutes. They hit all the combos I love—sweet and spicy, crunchy and creamy, and smoky and fresh. Along with the aforementioned margarita, I love to pair these with either tortilla chips and salsa and grilled corn, or black beans and cilantro-lime rice.

MANGO SALSA:

1½ cups diced mango

½ red bell pepper, deseeded and diced

1 jalapeño pepper, deseeded and minced

⅓ cup diced red onions

2 tablespoons chopped cilantro

Juice of ½ lime

Salt

TACOS:

2 tablespoons extra-virgin olive oil

1½ pounds cod or tilapia fillets

Blackening seasoning

1 avocado

Juice of ½ lime

Salt

8 corn tortillas

1 cup lightly packed shredded cabbage

1. In a medium bowl, mix together the mango, red pepper, jalapeño, red onions, and cilantro. Stir in the lime juice and season with a pinch of salt; set aside.

2. Heat the olive oil in a large nonstick skillet over medium-high heat. Sprinkle the fish generously with blackening seasoning; place in the skillet and cook until the fish flakes easily with a fork, 2 to 3 minutes per side. Remove and set aside.

3. While the fish is cooking, halve, peel, and pit the avocado; mash with the back of a fork, leaving it somewhat chunky. Stir in the lime juice and a pinch of salt.

4. Warm the tortillas over a gas flame until pliable and lightly charred. To assemble the tacos, spread each tortilla with a little avocado mash, then top each with 2 tablespoons of shredded cabbage, a few chunks of fish, and some mango salsa. Serve immediately.

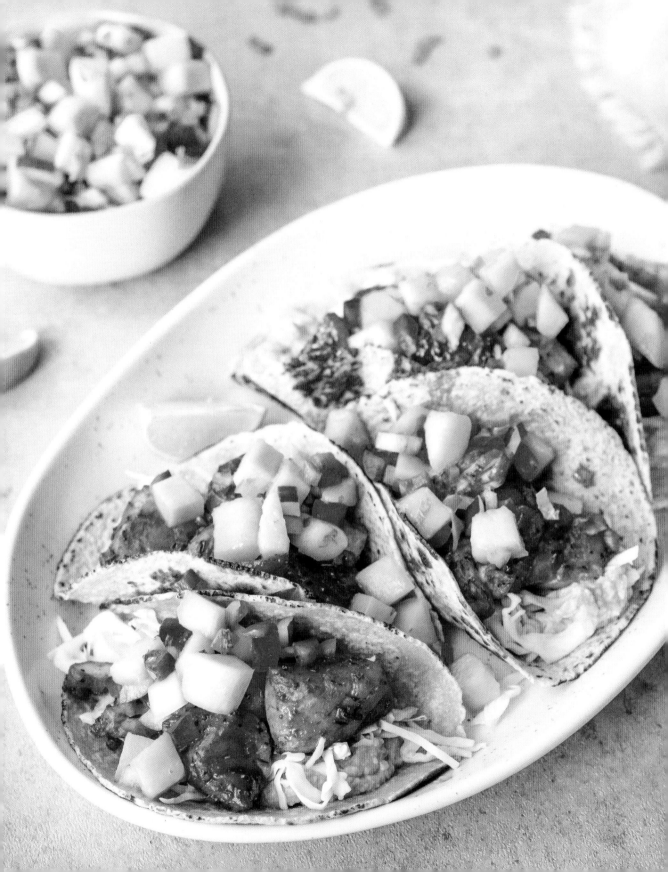

Cedar Plank Honey Mustard
TROUT WITH APPLE SALSA

——— MAKES 4 servings   PREP TIME: 15 minutes, plus time to soak cedar plank   COOK TIME: 25 minutes ———

When it comes to fatty fish, there are so many options beyond salmon. Trout is one of my favorites; it has a milder flavor. In fact, trout is often called "the chicken of the sea." It's perfect if you don't love the fishy taste of salmon but want to include more omega-3s in your diet. You may see a couple different kinds of trout at the grocery store: rainbow and steelhead. Rainbow trout has a mild taste, whereas steelhead has a richer, fattier flavor without being overly fishy. This recipe has you baste the trout in a tangy honey mustard sauce and cook it on a cedar plank, which smokes and flavors the fish. The tart apple salsa balances out the richness of the fish and adds a bit of crunch. Any leftover salsa is great as a snack with tortilla chips; just eat it within a day to prevent browning.

TROUT:

2 tablespoons honey

1½ tablespoons Dijon mustard

1½ tablespoons whole-grain mustard

Juice of ½ lemon

2 cloves garlic, minced

2 tablespoons thinly sliced chives, divided

Salt and black pepper

1 (1- to 1½-pound) trout fillet

SALSA:

1 Granny Smith or Golden Delicious apple, diced

1 avocado, diced

1 cup peeled, deseeded, and diced cucumbers

½ cup finely diced red onions

1 jalapeño pepper, deseeded and minced

Juice of ½ lemon

Salt

1. Turn on one burner of a gas grill, setting it to medium-high heat; leave the other burner off. (If you use a charcoal grill, light a chimney full of coals, wait until the coals are covered in a faint coat of white ash, and pile them on one side of the grill to create a two-zone fire, aiming for 375°F.)

2. While the grill is heating, whisk together the honey, mustards, lemon juice, garlic, and 1 tablespoon of the chives; season with salt and pepper. Pat the cedar plank dry and place the trout on it. Spread the sauce evenly over the trout.

3. Place the cedar plank with the trout on the area of the grill opposite the heat source. Close the lid and cook, checking every so often to make sure the plank isn't burning, until the fish flakes easily, 20 to 25 minutes. A thinner fillet will cook in less time, whereas a thicker fillet may take a bit longer.

4. While the fish is cooking, make the salsa: Mix together the apple, avocado, cucumbers, onions, jalapeño, and lemon juice; season with salt to taste.

5. Divide the trout into 4 servings. Top with a heaping scoop of the salsa and garnish with the remaining 1 tablespoon of chives.

SPECIAL EQUIPMENT:

Cedar plank about 14 by 7 inches, soaked in water for at least 2 hours

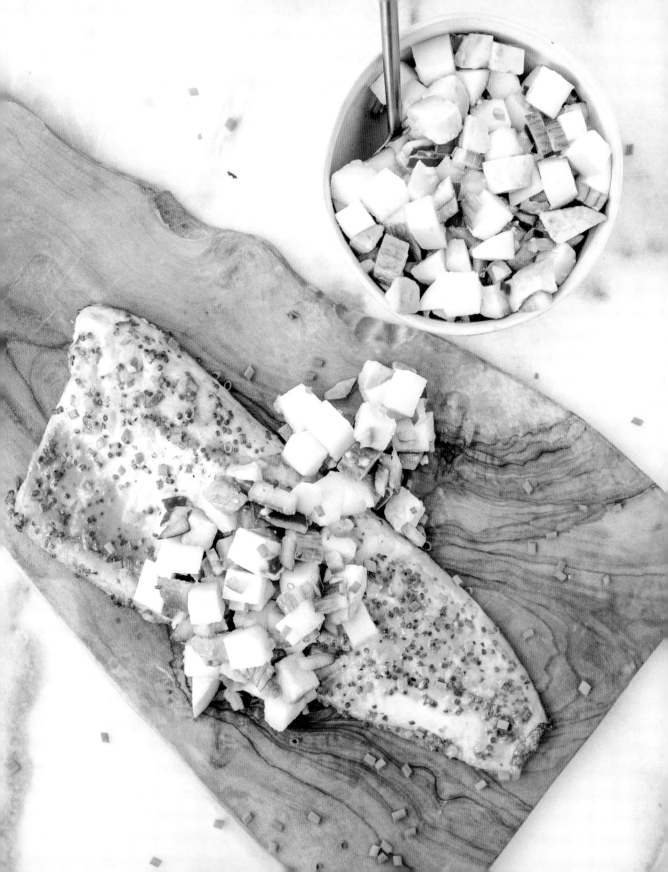

Mediterranean Chicken
HUMMUS BOWL

MAKES about 4 servings   PREP TIME: 15 minutes, plus time to marinate chicken and pickle onions
————————————————————— COOK TIME: 14 minutes —————————————————————

Turning hummus into a meal is a special skill of mine, and one of my favorite ways to do it is with a loaded hummus bowl. I've made countless variations, filling bowls of hummus with tasty ingredients like spice-roasted cauliflower and halloumi cheese and Israeli salad. I have even served shakshuka, a Mediterranean dish of eggs stewed in tomato sauce, in a well of garlicky hummus. Paired with some warm pita bread, it makes for one super satisfying meal. This version is filled with a sauté of chunks of garlicky chicken thighs with zucchini and cherry tomatoes and topped with all my favorite Mediterranean garnishes.

This recipe makes quite a bit more pickled red onions than you need, so there will be some left over. They're so delicious, you won't mind the extra. Store them in a mason jar and keep refrigerated for up to two weeks. You can use these pickled red onions to add a punch to grain bowls, tacos, salads, stir-fries, wraps, sautéed greens, grilled fish, curries—pretty much anything!

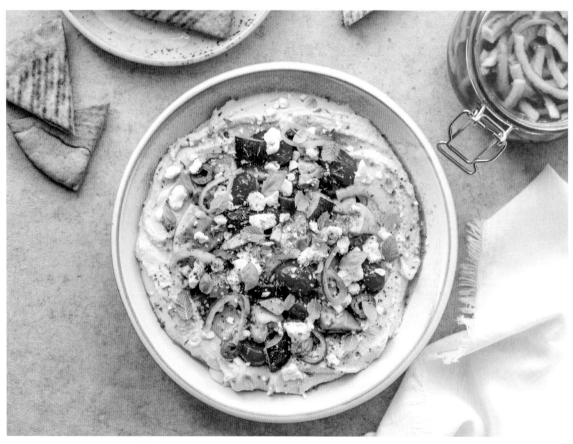

CHICKEN SAUTÉ:

Juice of 1 lemon

3 tablespoons extra-virgin olive oil, divided

2 cloves garlic, minced

½ teaspoon dried oregano

¼ teaspoon smoked paprika

¼ teaspoon salt

¼ teaspoon black pepper

1 pound boneless, skinless chicken thighs, cut into bite-sized chunks

1 large zucchini, cut into ¾-inch cubes

1½ cups cherry tomatoes

PICKLED RED ONIONS:

2 small red onions, halved lengthwise and sliced very thinly crosswise

2 teaspoons granulated sugar

2 teaspoons salt

2 cups warm water

1 cup apple cider vinegar

HUMMUS BOWL:

1½ cups hummus

¼ cup Kalamata olives, halved

¼ cup crumbled feta cheese

Chopped herbs, like mint, basil, or parsley, for serving (optional)

Pita bread, for serving

1. Marinate the chicken: In a large zip-top plastic bag or lidded container, whisk together the lemon juice, 2 tablespoons of the olive oil, the garlic, oregano, paprika, salt, and pepper. Add the chicken, toss to combine, and refrigerate for at least 1 hour. If making this recipe on a weeknight, this step, along with the pickled red onions in Step 2, can be done in the morning.

2. Prepare the pickled red onions: Place the onion slices in a quart-size mason jar. Dissolve the sugar and salt in the warm water. Stir in the vinegar. Pour over the onion slices, making sure they're fully submerged; refrigerate for at least 1 hour to pickle.

3. When ready to cook, preheat the oven to 350°F for toasting the pita. Heat the remaining 1 tablespoon of olive oil in a large skillet over medium-high heat. Add the zucchini and tomatoes and sauté until the vegetables start to soften, 3 to 4 minutes. Drain off and discard the marinade and add the chicken to the skillet. Sauté until the chicken is cooked through and the vegetables are tender, 7 to 10 minutes.

4. While the chicken and vegetables are cooking, toast the pita in the oven for a few minutes, until golden brown and crispy. Remove from the oven and cut into wedges.

5. Scoop the hummus into a large serving dish, making a well in the middle. Top with the chicken sauté. Sprinkle with the olives, feta, a few pickled onion slices, and herbs, if using, and serve with the toasted pita bread.

Lemon–Thyme Chicken with
PARMESAN ROASTED BROCCOLI & HERBED BROWN RICE

MAKES 3 to 4 servings   PREP TIME: 35 minutes   COOK TIME: 1 hour

I felt bad for ragging on the basic dieter's meal of chicken breast, broccoli, and brown rice so much in this book, so I decided to give it a gourmet makeover—because chicken breast, broccoli, and brown rice can actually taste good when pleasure is the goal. While I am partial to chicken thighs, boneless, skinless chicken breasts are really easy to cook and affordable, and this method of preparing them is my favorite. Simmering the breasts in the pan sauce keeps them juicy. The herbed brown rice in this recipe is pretty much the only way I prepare brown rice. Toasting the rice in oil brings out its nuttiness and helps prevent it from getting gummy, while the onion, garlic, and broth add tons of flavor. Lastly, there's the Parmesan roasted broccoli, which gets super crispy in the oven. It's the perfect recipe for making peace with chicken breast, broccoli, and brown rice.

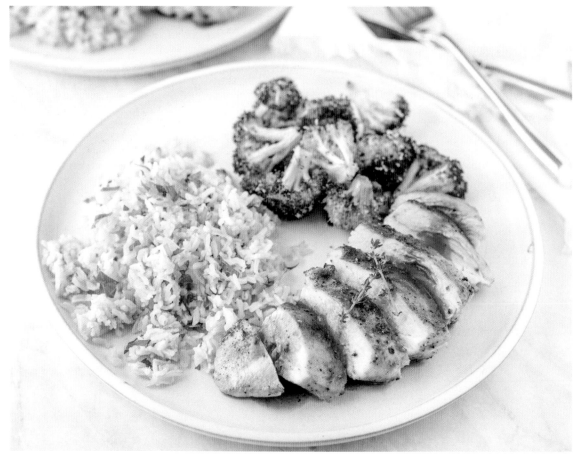

SEARED LEMON-THYME CHICKEN:

2 large boneless, skinless chicken breasts (about 1½ pounds total)

3 tablespoons extra-virgin olive oil, divided

¼ teaspoon paprika

¼ teaspoon garlic powder

¼ teaspoon onion powder

¼ teaspoon salt

¼ teaspoon black pepper

¾ cup low-sodium chicken or vegetable broth

¼ cup dry white wine

Juice of ½ lemon

2 sprigs thyme

HERBED BROWN RICE:

1 tablespoon extra-virgin olive oil

½ large yellow onion, chopped

Salt

1 clove garlic, minced

1 cup long-grain brown rice

2 cups low-sodium chicken or vegetable broth

2 tablespoons chopped parsley

PARMESAN ROASTED BROCCOLI:

1 head broccoli, cut into florets

2 tablespoons extra-virgin olive oil

½ cup grated Parmesan cheese

¼ teaspoon garlic powder

Pinch of red pepper flakes

1. Preheat the oven to 400°F.

2. Marinate the chicken: Pat the chicken dry with a paper towel. Place in a large zip-top plastic bag and lightly pound to flatten it out a bit. Drizzle with 1 tablespoon of the olive oil and mix in the paprika, garlic, onion powder, salt, and pepper; mix well. Leave to marinate for about 15 minutes.

3. Prepare the rice: Heat the olive oil in a medium saucepan over medium-high heat. Add the onion and a pinch of salt and cook, stirring occasionally, until the onion is translucent, about 5 minutes. Add the garlic and cook until fragrant, 30 seconds to 1 minute. Mix in the rice and cook, stirring frequently, until the rice is slightly translucent, about 2 minutes. Pour in the broth and bring to a boil. Reduce the heat, cover, and simmer until the broth is absorbed, 40 to 50 minutes. Let the rice sit, covered, for 5 to 10 minutes to finish steaming. Fluff with a fork and stir in the parsley.

4. While the rice is cooking, roast the broccoli: Toss the broccoli with the olive oil, Parmesan, and garlic powder. Spread evenly on a sheet pan lined with parchment pepper and roast, flipping halfway through cooking, until golden brown and crispy, about 30 minutes.

5. Cook the chicken: Heat the remaining 2 tablespoons of olive oil in a large nonstick skillet over medium-high heat. Add the chicken breasts and cook without moving until it has a nice seared crust, 5 to 7 minutes. Turn the chicken over and pour the broth, wine, lemon juice, and thyme into the skillet. Reduce the heat to medium, cover, and simmer until the chicken is cooked through, 6 to 8 minutes.

6. Remove the chicken to a clean plate and let it rest for 5 minutes. Increase the heat under the skillet to medium-high and simmer the pan sauce to reduce it by half, 2 to 3 minutes.

7. Slice the chicken on the diagonal and serve drizzled with the pan sauce alongside the brown rice and roasted broccoli.

One-Pan Harissa
CHICKEN & RICE

— MAKES 4 servings   PREP TIME: 20 minutes   COOK TIME: 45 minutes —

This one-pan meal combines spicy, smoky chicken thighs and perfectly cooked rice with bold Moroccan flavors. If you've been running through the same boring weeknight chicken recipes, you'll love this dish! My favorite type of chicken to cook is skin-on chicken thighs. With a bit more fat and lots more flavor, I find them to be much juicier and more satisfying than the breasts. Remember, even though diet culture elevates chicken breasts, fat is nothing to fear. If you enjoy chicken thighs, eat them!

4 bone-in, skin-on chicken thighs

4 tablespoons extra-virgin olive oil, divided

2 tablespoons store-bought harissa

Salt

1 large yellow onion, finely diced

4 cloves garlic, minced

1 teaspoon ground cumin

½ teaspoon ground coriander

⅛ teaspoon ground cinnamon

2 cardamom pods, or a pinch of ground cardamom

1 cup basmati rice

1 (15-ounce) can chickpeas, drained and rinsed

⅓ cup golden raisins

⅓ cup chopped green olives

Grated zest and juice of ½ lemon

1½ cups low-sodium chicken or vegetable broth

½ teaspoon salt

¼ teaspoon cracked black pepper

¼ cup roughly chopped raw almonds

1 tablespoon chopped mint, for garnish

1 tablespoon chopped parsley, for garnish

1. Preheat the oven to 425°F.

2. In a large mixing bowl, rub the chicken thighs with 1 tablespoon of the olive oil, the harissa, and a large pinch of salt; set aside.

3. Heat the remaining 3 tablespoons of olive oil in a large ovenproof skillet over medium-high heat. Add the onion and a pinch of salt and cook, stirring occasionally, until lightly golden. Stir in the garlic and cook until fragrant, about 1 minute. Stir in the cumin, coriander, cinnamon, and cardamom pods and cook for 30 seconds. Add the rice and cook for 1 minute, stirring constantly. Turn off the heat. Stir in the chickpeas, raisins, olives, lemon zest and juice, broth, salt, and pepper.

4. Nestle the marinated chicken thighs into the rice mixture. Sprinkle the almonds on top. Bake until the chicken is golden brown and the juices run clear, 40 to 45 minutes. Let cool for 5 minutes. Serve garnished with mint and parsley. (You can remove and discard the cardamom pods or leave them in to keep the dish fragrant; just don't eat them.)

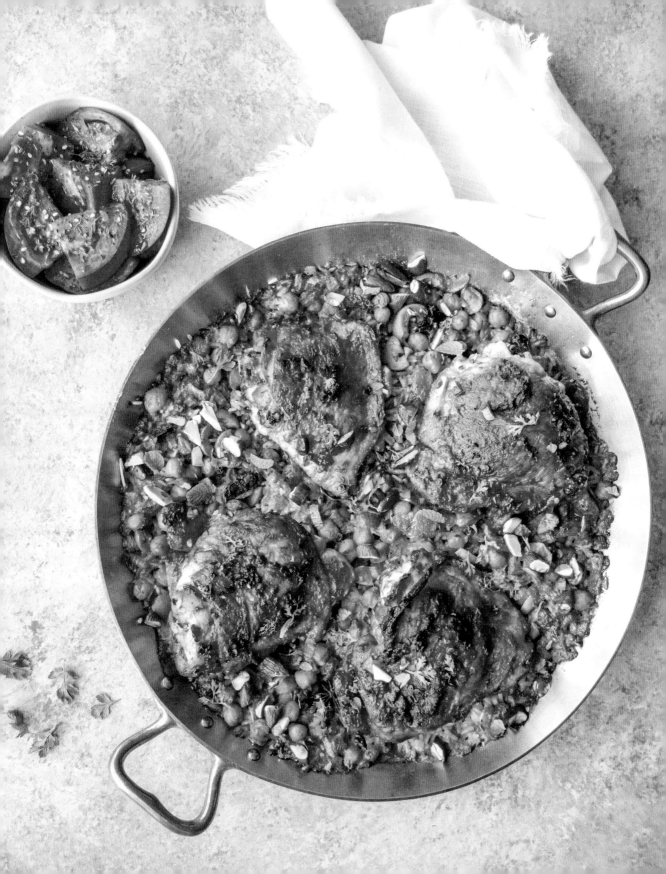

Shepherd's Pie with
HERBED POTATO TOPPING

MAKES 4 servings   PREP TIME: 25 minutes   COOK TIME: 1 hour

Shepherd's pie is a classic comfort food, with a layer of ground beef and vegetables simmered in a flavorful sauce, topped with creamy mashed potatoes. This recipe gets a few flavor upgrades, with mashed potatoes flecked with herbs and topped with Parmesan and finely diced mushrooms—my secret flavor booster—mixed with the beef for an even meatier flavor. In fact, if you prefer, you can even replace some of the ground beef with more of the "mushroom meat."

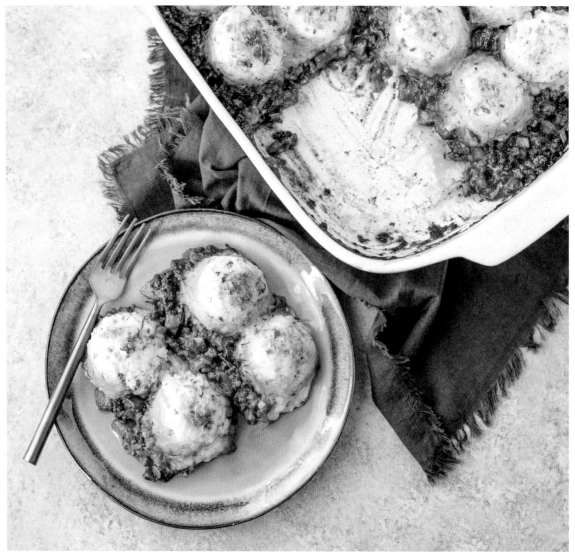

MASHED POTATO TOPPING:

2 pounds Yukon Gold potatoes, peeled if desired, cut into 1-inch cubes

2 tablespoons unsalted butter

½ cup whole or 2% milk

2 tablespoons chopped chives or scallions

2 tablespoons chopped dill

2 tablespoons chopped parsley

Salt and black pepper

⅓ cup grated Parmesan cheese

FILLING:

2 tablespoons extra-virgin olive oil

1 large yellow onion, diced

8 ounces cremini mushrooms, diced

2 medium carrots, halved lengthwise and sliced into ¼-inch pieces

2 celery stalks, chopped

4 cloves garlic, minced

Leaves from 3 sprigs thyme

2 bay leaves

Salt and black pepper

1 pound ground beef

1 tablespoon tomato paste

⅓ cup dry red wine

1 tablespoon soy sauce

2 tablespoons all-purpose flour

1 cup low-sodium beef broth

1. Put the potatoes in a large pot and cover with a couple inches of salted water. Bring to a boil and cook until tender, about 10 minutes. Drain and return the cooked potatoes to the pot. Add the butter and milk and mash until combined and smooth. Stir in the chives, dill, and parsley and season to taste with salt and pepper.

2. Preheat the oven to 400°F.

3. Prepare the filling: Heat the olive oil in a 4-quart Dutch oven over medium-high heat. Add the onion, mushrooms, carrots, celery, garlic, thyme, and bay leaves, along with a pinch of salt and pepper; cook until the onion is translucent and the vegetables are tender, about 10 minutes.

4. Add the ground beef and cook, breaking the beef apart with a spatula, until no pink remains, about 5 minutes. Stir in the tomato paste and cook for 1 minute longer. Add the wine and soy sauce, scraping up the browned bits at the bottom, and cook until the liquid is mostly absorbed, about 2 minutes.

5. Stir in the flour, cook for a minute, and then pour in the broth. Bring to a simmer and cook until slightly thickened, about 5 minutes. Remove and discard the bay leaves.

6. Transfer the beef filling to a 9 by 11-inch casserole dish, leveling the top with a spatula. Using an ice cream scoop, scoop the mashed potatoes over the top of the filling. Sprinkle the tops of the potatoes with the Parmesan cheese.

7. Bake the pie until the filling is bubbly and the potatoes are lightly golden, 20 to 25 minutes. Let cool for 5 minutes before serving.

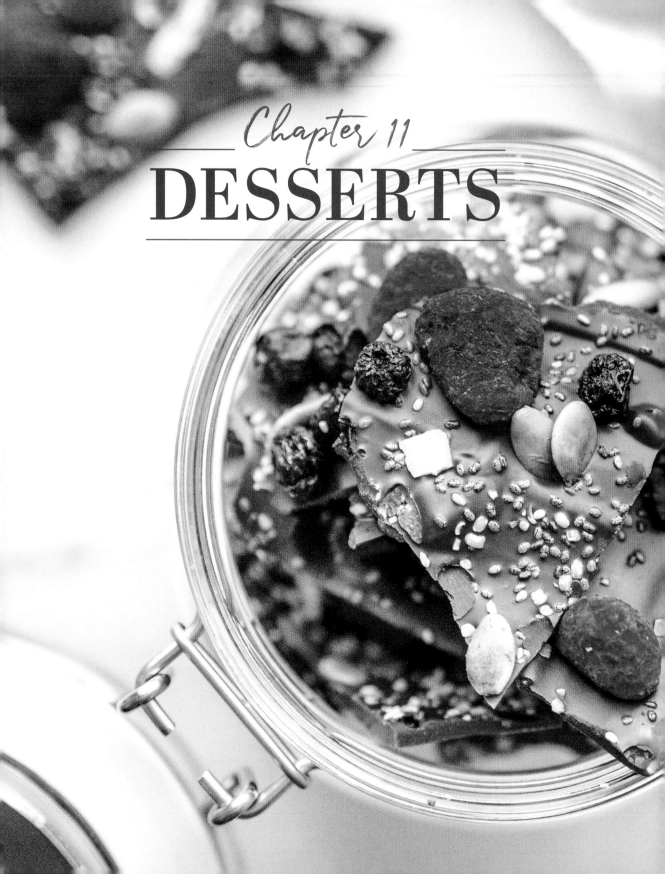

Chapter 11
DESSERTS

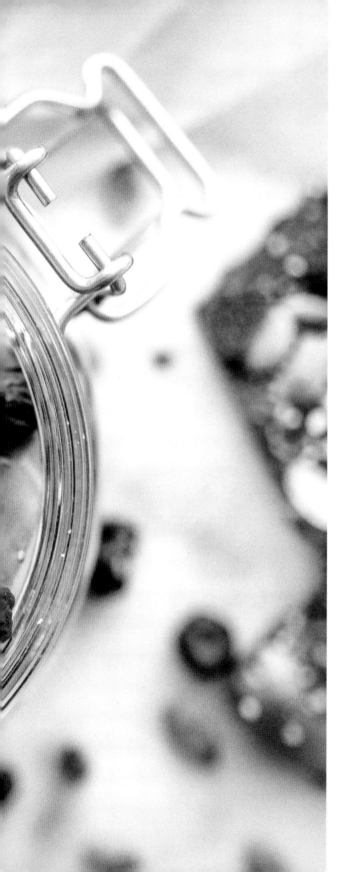

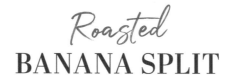

Roasted BANANA SPLIT

MAKES 1 serving   PREP TIME: 10 minutes   COOK TIME: 20 minutes

Fruit for dessert? No, thanks. Whenever I read diet advice to eat fruit for dessert, my eyes roll so far back in my head that I'm surprised they've never gotten stuck there. With a few exceptions, like when a fruit is perfectly ripe and in season (hello, South Carolina peaches!), fruit for dessert just isn't satisfying to me. Fruit in dessert, however, is a different story. Roasting concentrates the sweetness of bananas and gives them a luxurious texture. And while I'm rarely a fruit-for-dessert person, I often make these roasted bananas and enjoy them on their own. Topping this split with coconut milk ice cream and shredded coconut gives it a tropical flair. This dessert tastes like how sunscreen smells, and I mean that in the best possible way!

1 banana

1 tablespoon salted butter, cut into 6 pieces

1 scoop coconut milk ice cream or coconut-flavored ice cream

FOR GARNISH:

Chopped dark chocolate

Unsweetened shredded coconut

Chopped roasted pistachios

1. Preheat the oven to 400°F. Line a sheet pan with parchment paper.

2. Carefully halve the banana lengthwise. Place the halves cut side up on the prepared pan. Put 3 pieces of butter on each half. Roast until lightly golden and tender, about 20 minutes.

3. Transfer the roasted banana to a serving bowl. Top with a scoop of ice cream and garnish with chocolate, shredded coconut, and pistachios.

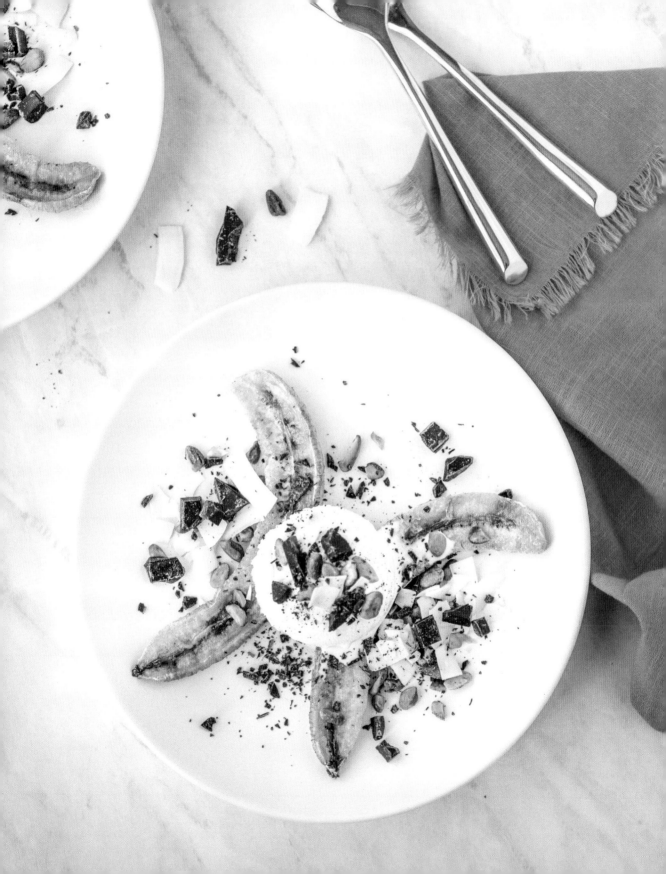

Almond Chocolate
CHUNK COOKIES

MAKES 24 to 28 cookies PREP TIME: 10 minutes COOK TIME: 30 minutes

Chocolate chip cookies are my go-to when it comes to comfort baking, procrasti-baking, or I-need-something-sweet-but-there's-nothing-in-the-house baking. I honestly don't think there is a more perfect dessert than a freshly baked chocolate chip cookie, except for maybe tiramisu (but that takes much more time and many more ingredients). I've been playing around with various cookie recipes for the past few years, and one thing I've discovered is that I love the addition of almond meal. When used in a 50/50ish mix with all-purpose flour, it gives cookies an incredible nutty flavor and a pleasantly crumbly texture. Thanks to the popularity of gluten-free, Paleo, and keto diets, almond meal has become hugely popular. While I appreciate that it is getting some love, I don't appreciate that it has been claimed by diet culture. I use it as a way to add flavor and texture instead of as a way to avoid gluten or carbs. Besides cookies, I love to use almond meal in banana bread and in muffins and as a crumb topping for casseroles. It also makes a tasty crust for pan-fried seafood, especially when combined with panko.

---

1 cup (2 sticks) unsalted butter, at room temperature

¾ cup packed brown sugar

⅓ cup granulated sugar

⅓ cup almond butter

1 large egg, at room temperature

2 teaspoons vanilla extract

½ teaspoon almond extract

1¼ cups all-purpose flour

1 cup almond meal

½ teaspoon baking soda

½ teaspoon fine sea salt

1½ cups chopped dark chocolate–covered almonds

Flaky sea salt, for sprinkling

1. Preheat the oven to 350°F. Line a baking sheet with parchment paper.

2. In a large mixing bowl, beat the butter and sugars using a hand mixer (or use a stand mixer fitted with the paddle attachment) on high speed until fluffy. Beat in the almond butter, egg, and extracts until creamy. Add the flour, almond meal, baking soda, and fine salt; beat on medium speed until combined. Stir in the chocolate-covered almonds.

3. Scoop tablespoonfuls of the dough, roll into balls, and arrange the balls 2 inches apart on the prepared baking sheet. Sprinkle with the flaky salt.

4. Bake for 8 minutes. Remove the baking sheet from the oven and tap it on the counter a few times to flatten the cookies. Place the sheet back in the oven and bake until the cookies are set on the edges but still a bit doughy in the middle, 1 to 2 minutes. Let cool on the pan for a few minutes before transferring to a cooling rack to cool completely.

5. Repeat with the remaining dough, making a total of 24 to 28 cookies. Store in an airtight container at room temperature for up to 5 days.

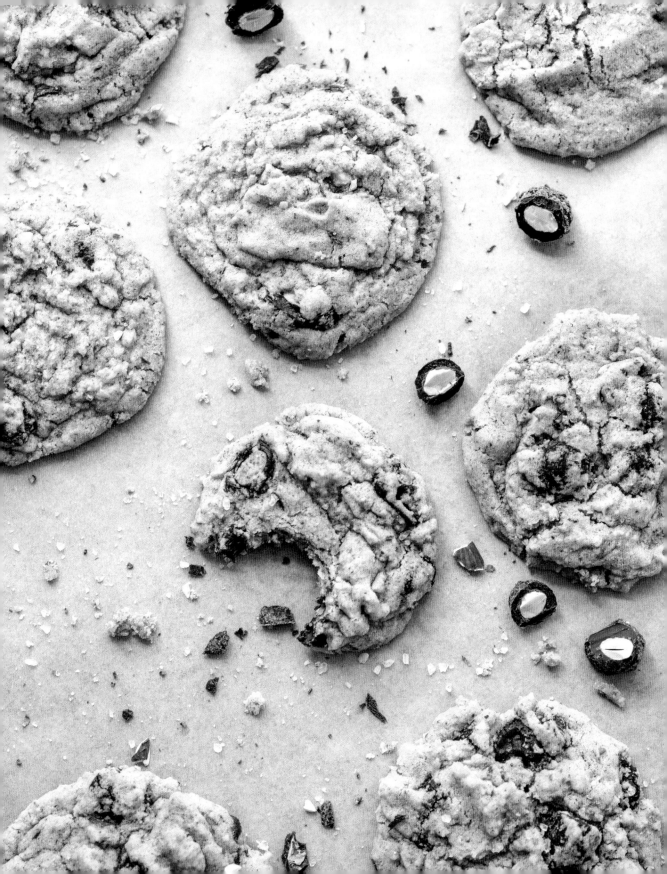

Seedy Dark Chocolate
BARK WITH BERRIES

MAKES about 30 pieces   PREP TIME: 10 minutes, plus 30 minutes to chill   COOK TIME: 2 minutes

A common taste hunger is the desire for something sweet after dinner. Sometimes the taste hunger is for a more substantial dessert. Other times you just want the flavor of something sweet to finish off a meal. This dark chocolate bark is perfect for the latter scenario. Melting coconut oil with semisweet chocolate chips makes the bark taste luxurious and gives it a smooth, melt-in-the-mouth consistency. It's a way to turn a basic bag of chocolate chips into "gourmet" chocolate. The freeze-dried berries and the seeds add a bit of tart flavor and crunch; they also just look really pretty. (Hey, we eat with our eyes too!) You want to treat this recipe like an art project. Sprinkle on the freeze-dried berries and the pumpkin, hemp, and chia seeds in the amounts that you like and in a way that looks pretty to you.

1 (12-ounce) bag semisweet chocolate chips

2 tablespoons coconut oil

A couple handfuls of freeze-dried berries

A handful of pumpkin seeds

2 tablespoons hemp hearts

1 tablespoon chia seeds

1. Line a baking sheet with parchment paper. Make enough room in the refrigerator for the baking sheet to lie flat on a shelf.

2. Put the chocolate chips and coconut oil in a large microwave-safe bowl. Microwave on high in 20-second increments, stirring after each, until smooth and homogenous.

3. Use a spatula to spread the melted chocolate evenly into a ¼-inch-thick layer on the prepared baking sheet.

4. Sprinkle the freeze-dried berries, pumpkin seeds, hemp hearts, and chia seeds on top of the chocolate. Place the sheet in the refrigerator and chill until the chocolate is set, about 30 minutes.

5. Break the bark into pieces. Store in a lidded container in the refrigerator for up to 2 weeks.

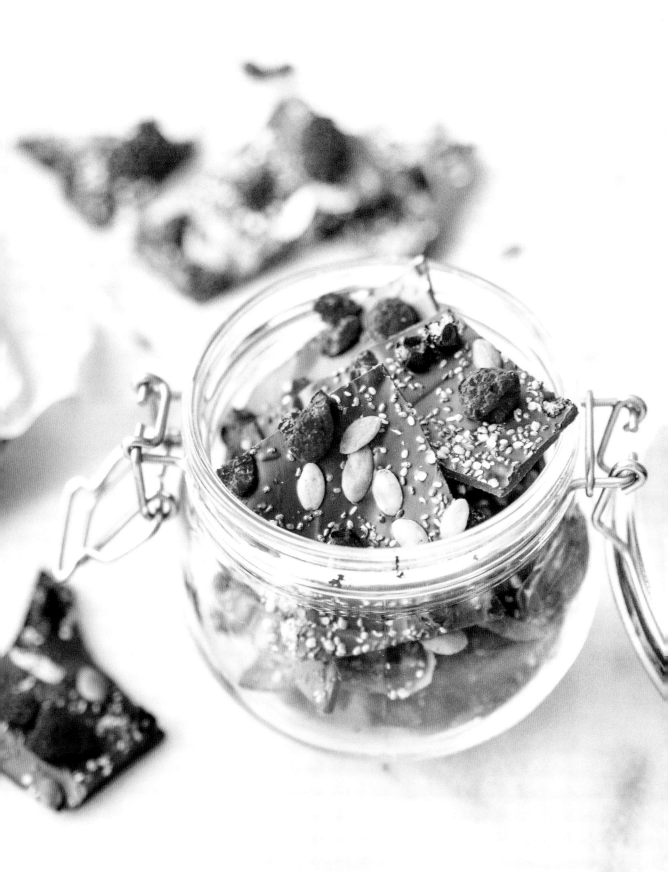

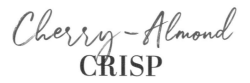

Cherry–Almond CRISP

———— MAKES 6 servings PREP TIME: 15 minutes COOK TIME: 50 minutes ————

Most "healthy" dessert recipes force in fruits and whole grains in the form of ingredient swaps, like using mashed banana in lieu of butter (ick) or all whole-grain flours in a cake (also ick). Crisps, cobblers, and crumbles are examples of how those nutrient-rich ingredients can naturally be a part of desserts, adding flavor rather than subtracting.

This cherry-almond crisp couldn't be easier to make. Just top a couple bags of frozen fruit with a crumble made from kitchen staples. This recipe can be made with any frozen fruit you like—peaches, blueberries, and strawberries work particularly well. My favorite way to enjoy this crisp is with a scoop of mascarpone drizzled with honey, but you can't go wrong with a scoop of classic vanilla ice cream. Leftover crisp is delicious for breakfast, served over Greek yogurt. In fact, I often bake a crisp specifically to enjoy for breakfast!

If you must avoid gluten, feel free to swap in gluten-free baking flour; this recipe works very well with almond meal as well. I've also made it with coconut oil when I was out of butter, and it worked really well too, imparting a subtle coconut flavor to the topping.

FILLING:

2 (16-ounce) bags frozen cherries

2 tablespoons packed brown sugar

2 teaspoons cornstarch

1 teaspoon vanilla extract

Pinch of salt

TOPPING:

½ cup (1 stick) unsalted butter, melted

1 cup rolled oats

½ cup whole-wheat flour

½ cup all-purpose flour

⅓ cup roughly chopped raw almonds

¼ cup packed brown sugar

1 teaspoon vanilla extract

¼ teaspoon salt

1. Preheat the oven to 375°F.

2. Make the filling: In a 9 by 11-inch baking dish, stir together the cherries, brown sugar, cornstarch, vanilla extract, and salt.

3. Make the topping: In a large bowl, use your hands to mix together the melted butter, oats, flours, almonds, brown sugar, vanilla extract, and salt until clumps form. Crumble the topping evenly over the cherry filling.

4. Bake until the cherries are bubbling and the topping is golden, 45 to 50 minutes.

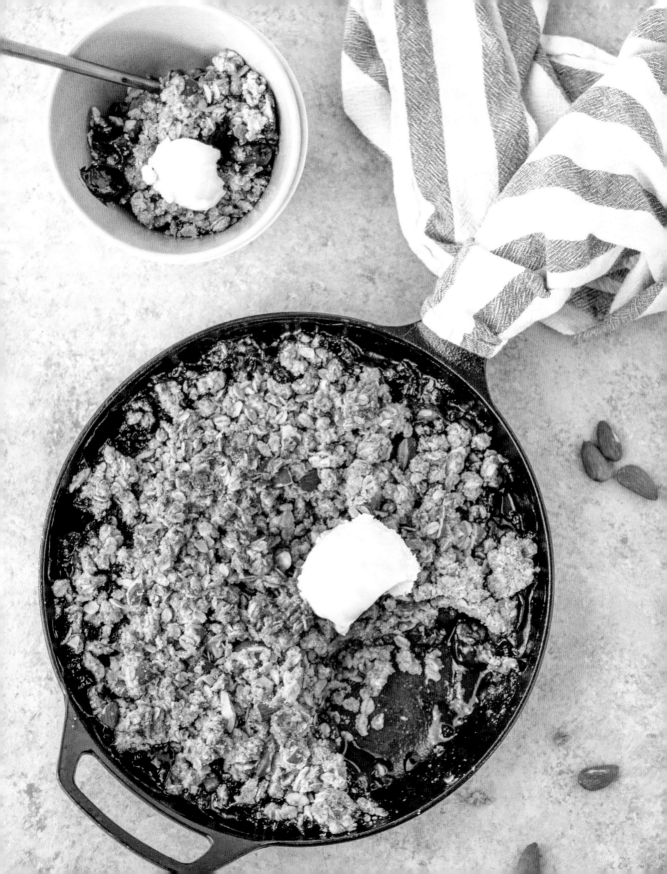

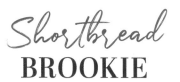

Shortbread
BROOKIE

MAKES 24 bars   PREP TIME: 20 minutes   COOK TIME: 65 minutes

Sometimes the healthiest thing you can eat is a really good brownie. If there's one takeaway from this book, it's that healthy eating is about more than nutrition. While a brownie might not provide your body with its daily needs for vitamin A or a whole bunch of fiber, it nourishes you in other ways. This shortbread brookie of dense, fudgy brownie with a perfectly crackly top, baked over a chocolate chip shortbread crust, is a favorite of mine.

SHORTBREAD CRUST:

¾ cup (1½ sticks) unsalted butter, at room temperature

1½ cups all-purpose flour

¼ cup granulated sugar

½ teaspoon salt

⅓ cup semisweet chocolate chips

BROWNIE LAYER:

1 cup (2 sticks) unsalted butter, at room temperature

1½ cups semisweet chocolate chips

1½ cups granulated sugar

1 tablespoon vanilla extract

½ cup all-purpose flour

½ cup unsweetened cocoa powder

1 teaspoon baking powder

½ teaspoon salt

4 large eggs, at room temperature

Flaky sea salt, for sprinkling

1. Preheat the oven to 350°F. Grease a 9 by 13-inch baking dish.

2. Make the crust: In a food processor, pulse the butter, flour, sugar, and salt, scraping down the sides as needed. When combined, add the chocolate chips and pulse a few times until the chips are chopped in. The dough should form small chunks resembling the pieces of chocolate chip cookie dough in ice cream.

3. Press the shortbread dough into the greased baking dish to form a crust. Prick all over with a fork. Bake until lightly browned, about 30 minutes.

4. Meanwhile, prepare the brownie layer: Put the butter and chocolate chips in a large microwave-safe bowl and microwave in 30-second increments, stirring after each, until smooth and homogenous. Stir in the sugar and vanilla extract.

5. In a separate medium bowl, whisk together the flour, cocoa powder, baking powder, and salt; set aside.

6. In a third bowl, whisk the eggs until frothy, about a minute. Stir the whisked eggs into the chocolate and butter mixture. Add the dry ingredients and stir until combined.

7. Spread the brownie batter evenly over the shortbread crust and sprinkle the flaky salt on top. Bake until the brownie layer is just set, about 35 minutes. Let cool and cut into bars before serving.

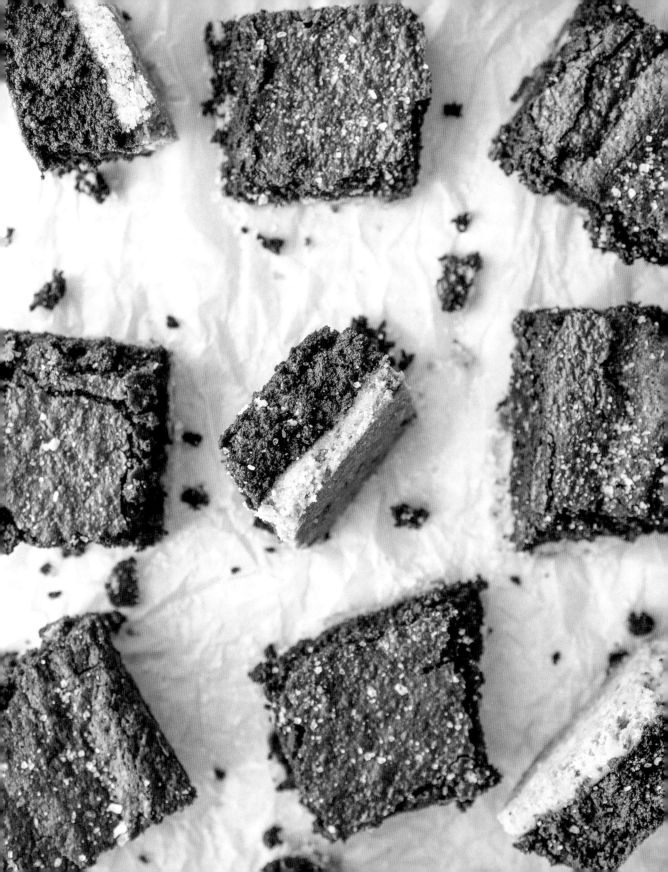

Acknowledgments

This book would not exist without the work of the many, many non-diet dietitians, fat activists, and Health at Every Size researchers before me who have informed my work over the years. Non-diet approaches to health and nutrition should be the standard and yet, as anyone who has worked in this field knows, are actually radical and can often feel like swimming upstream in this diet culture we all live in. I want to specifically thank Evelyn Tribole and Elyse Resch whose book, *Intuitive Eating,* first gave me the language to practice with a non-diet approach, as well as Lindo Bacon, Lucy Aphramor, Regan Chastain, Sonya Renee Taylor, Christy Harrison, Marci Evans, Kelsey Miller, and Aubrey Gordon of Your Fat Friend whose work has been most influential to me. An extra dose of gratitude goes to Anna Sweeney for your mentorship and friendship and for being the only person I know who can almost choke to death laughing over an eggplant.

To Kara, Meme, Min, Marisa, Alex, Anne, Alexis, Robyn, Kylie, and Haley—you have become friends as much as colleagues over the years. When I say I couldn't have written this book without you, I truly mean it. I felt lost in the wilderness in those early days of starting my own practice, and I could not have made it through without your support and advice.

Thank you to my team at Victory Belt, for dealing with my insecure writer's anxiety, and also believing in me, and this book. A massive thank you to my editor, Siri, for all the care and consideration you put into each word in this book.

To my family and friends—I am endlessly grateful to you for your love and support. The way you have celebrated, shared, and uplifted my work has meant the world to me. When we can safely gather again, I promise to throw a big launch party at our house with plenty of cheese and wine and hugs and thank each one of you!

To Scott—I honestly don't know if I have the words to express my gratitude. Thank you for believing in me when I didn't believe in myself and for always reminding me of my successes when my anxious brain was wrapped up in my failures. Thank you for only complaining a little bit about the number of dishes in the sink after a long day of recipe testing or the last-minute trips to the grocery store every time I ran out of onions. I love you so, so much.

And finally, to my clients—I am endlessly grateful for the trust you put in me by sharing with me your story and allowing me to be part of your journey. You have been my greatest teachers, and this book would not exist without you.

About the Author

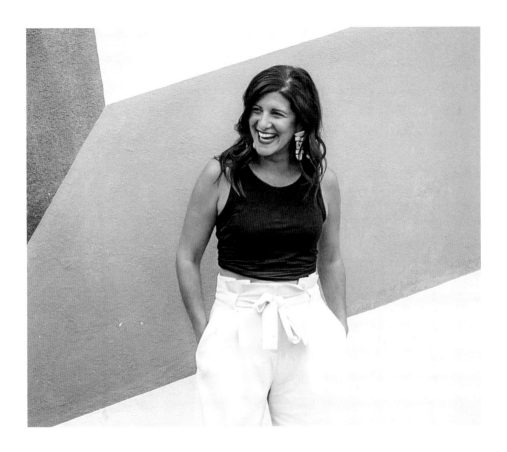

Rachael Hartley, RD, LD, is a Columbia, SC-based nutrition therapist, certified intuitive eating counselor, and a food and nutrition expert who is featured regularly in national media. Passionate about helping others rediscover the joy of eating and foster a healthier relationship with food, she founded Rachael Hartley Nutrition, a weight-inclusive practice where she specializes in women's health, disordered eating, and healing from chronic dieting, IBS, and other digestive disorders. In addition to her practice and conducting presentations on intuitive eating and non-diet nutrition to both professional audiences and the general public, Rachael also runs the popular blog, *The Joy of Eating*, where she shares practical intuitive eating advice and non-diet recipes.

Notes

1 Linda Bacon et al., "Size Acceptance and Intuitive Eating Improve Health for Obese, Female Chronic Dieters," *Journal of the American Dietetic Association* 105, no. 6 (2005): 929–36.

2 Janell Mensinger and Heather A. Yarger, "Intuitive Eating: A Novel Health Promotion Strategy for Obese Women" (paper, 137th American Public Health Association Annual Meeting and Exposition, Philadelphia, PA, November 2009).

3 Dawn Clifford et al., "Impact of Non-Diet Approaches on Attitudes, Behaviors, and Health Outcomes: A Systematic Review," *Journal of Nutrition Education and Behavior* 47, no. 2 (2015): 144–55.e1.

4 Julie T. Schaefer and Amy B. Magnuson, "A Review of Interventions That Promote Eating by Internal Cues," *Journal of the Academy of Nutrition and Dietetics* 114, no. 5 (2014): 734–60.

5 Katherine M. Flegal et al., "Excess Deaths Associated with Underweight, Overweight, and Obesity," *Journal of the American Medical Association* 293, no. 15 (2005): 1861–7.

6 Paula M. Lantz et al., "Socioeconomic and Behavioral Risk Factors for Mortality in a National 19-Year Prospective Study of U.S. Adults," *Social Science & Medicine* 70, no. 10 (2010): 1558–66.

7 Alison Fildes et al., "Probability of an Obese Person Attaining Normal Body Weight: Cohort Study Using Electronic Health Records," *American Journal of Public Health* 105, no. 9 (2015): e54–9.

8 Laurie M. Anderson et al., "The Effectiveness of Worksite Nutrition and Physical Activity Interventions for Controlling Employee Overweight and Obesity," *American Journal of Preventive Medicine* 37, no. 4 (2009): 340–57.

9 Traci Mann et al., "Medicare's Search for Effective Obesity Treatments: Diets Are Not the Answer," *American Psychologist* 62, no. 3 (2007): 220–33.

10 Morten Nordmo, Yngvild Sørebø Danielsen, and Magnus Nordmo, "The Challenge of Keeping It Off: A Descriptive Systematic Review of High-Quality, Follow-Up Studies of Obesity Treatments," *Obesity Reviews* 21 (2020): e129–49.

11 Janet Tomiyama, Britt Ahlstrom, and Traci Mann, "Long-Term Effects of Dieting: Is Weight Loss Related to Health?" *Social and Personality Psychology Compass* 7, no. 12 (2013): 861–77.

12 Sandra Aamodt, "Why Dieting Doesn't Usually Work," filmed June 2013 in Edinburgh, TED video, 12:19, https://www.ted.com/talks/sandra_aamodt_why_dieting_doesn_t_usually_work?language=en.

13 Eric Doucet et al., "Relation Between Appetite Ratings Before and After a Standard Meal and Estimates of Daily Energy Intake in Obese and Reduced Obese Individuals," *Appetite* 40, no. 2 (2003): 137–43.

14 Priya Sumithran et al., "Long-Term Persistence of Hormonal Adaptations to Weight Loss," *New England Journal of Medicine* 365, no. 17 (2011): 1597–604.

15 Erin Fothergill et al., "Persistent Metabolic Adaptation 6 Years After 'The Biggest Loser' Competition," *Obesity* 24, no. 8 (2016): 1612–9.

16 David Polidori et al., "How Strongly Does Appetite Counter Weight Loss? Quantification of the Feedback Control of Human Energy Intake," *Obesity* 24, no. 11 (2016): 2289–95.

17 Leah M. Kalm and Richard D. Semba, "They Starved So That Others Be Better Fed: Remembering Ancel Keys and the Minnesota Experiment," *Journal of Nutrition* 135, no. 6 (2005): 1347–52.

18 Marie Galmiche et al., "Prevalence of Eating Disorders Over the 2000–2018 Period: A Systematic Literature Review," *American Journal of Clinical Nutrition* 109, no. 5 (2019): 1402–13.

19 Virgie Tovar, "Take The Cake: 8 Clues Your 'Lifestyle' Is Actually a Diet (& Why It's Gaslighting)," *Ravishly*, February 8, 2018, https://ravishly.com/lifestyle-actually-diet.

20 S. M. Phelan et al., "Impact of Weight Bias and Stigma on Quality of Care and Outcomes for Patients with Obesity," *Obesity Reviews* 16, no. 4 (2015): 319–26.

21 E. M. Matheson, D. E. King, and C. J. Everett, "Healthy Lifestyle Habits and Mortality in Overweight and Obese Individuals," *Journal of the American Board of Family Medicine* 25, no. 1 (2012): 9–15.

22 Tracy L. Tylka et al., "The Weight-Inclusive Versus Weight-Normative Approach to Health: Evaluating the Evidence for Prioritizing Well-Being over Weight Loss," *Journal of Obesity* 2014 (2014): 1–18.

23 Katharina Timper and Jens C. Brüning, "Hypothalamic Circuits Regulating Appetite and Energy Homeostasis: Pathways to Obesity," *Disease Models & Mechanisms* 10, no. 6 (2017): 679–89.

24 Vipul Periwal and Carson C. Chow, "Patterns in Food Intake Correlate with Body Mass Index," *American Journal of Physiology-Endocrinology and Metabolism* 291, no. 5 (2006): E929–36.

25 David C. Frankenfield, "Bias and Accuracy of Resting Metabolic Rate Equations in Non-Obese and Obese Adults," *Clinical Nutrition* 32, no. 6 (2013): 976–82.

26 "Guidance for Industry: Guide for Developing and Using Data Bases for Nutrition Labeling," *U.S. Food and Drug Administration*, published March 1998, https://www.fda.gov/regulatory-information/search-fda-guidance-documents/guidance-industry-guide-developing-and-using-data-bases-nutrition-labeling.

27 Janet A. Novotny, Sarah K. Gebauer, and David J. Baer, "Discrepancy Between the Atwater Factor Predicted and Empirically Measured Energy Values of Almonds in Human Diets," *American Journal of Clinical Nutrition* 96, no. 2 (2012): 296–301.

28 Maggie L. Zou et al., "Accuracy of the Atwater Factors and Related Food Energy Conversion Factors with Low-Fat, High-Fiber Diets When Energy Intake Is Reduced Spontaneously," *American Journal of Clinical Nutrition* 86, no. 6 (2007): 1649–56.

29 Armghan H. Ans et al., "Neurohormonal Regulation of Appetite and Its Relationship with Stress: A Mini Literature Review," *Cureus* 10, no. 7 (2018): e3032.

30 David R. Broom et al., "Influence of Resistance and Aerobic Exercise on Hunger, Circulating Levels of Acylated Ghrelin, and Peptide YY in Healthy Males," *American Journal of Physiology-Regulatory, Integrative and Comparative Physiology* 296, no. 1 (2009): R29–36.

31 Rachel D. Barnes and Stacey Tantleff-Dunn, "Food for Thought: Examining the Relationship Between Food Thought Suppression and Weight-Related Outcomes," *Eating Behaviors* 11, no. 3 (2010): 175–9.

32 Anna Richard et al., "Effects of Chocolate Deprivation on Implicit and Explicit Evaluation of Chocolate in High and Low Trait Chocolate Cravers," *Frontiers in Psychology* 8 (2017): 1591.

33 Leonard H. Epstein et al., "Habituation as a Determinant of Human Food Intake," *Psychological Review* 116, no. 2 (2009): 384–407.

34 Jeffrey M. Brunstrom and Gemma L. Mitchell, "Effects of Distraction on the Development of Satiety," *British Journal of Nutrition* 96, no. 4 (2006): 761–9.

35 Margaret L. Westwater, Paul C. Fletcher, and Hisham Ziauddeen, "Sugar Addiction: The State of the Science," *European Journal of Nutrition* 55, no. S2 (2016): 55–69.

36 *Ibid.*

37 Delores A. Smitham, "Evaluating an Intuitive Eating Program for Binge Eating Disorder: A Benchmarking Study" (PhD diss., University of Notre Dame, 2008).

38 Robert Ross and Ian Janssen, "Physical Activity, Total and Regional Obesity: Dose-Response Considerations," *Medicine and Science in Sports and Exercise* 33, 6 Suppl. (2001): S521–7.

39 Timothy S. Church et al., "Changes in Weight, Waist Circumference and Compensatory Responses with Different Doses of Exercise Among Sedentary, Overweight Postmenopausal Women," *PLoS ONE* 4, no. 2 (2009): e4515.

40 E. E. Hill et al., "Exercise and Circulating Cortisol Levels: The Intensity Threshold Effect," *Journal of Endocrinological Investigation* 31, no. 7 (2008): 587–91.

41 Philippe Vandenbroeck, Jo Goossens, and Marshall Clemens, "Obesity System Influence Diagram," *VisualComplexity*, accessed March 11, 2020, http://www.visualcomplexity.com/vc/project.cfm?id=622&fbclid=IwAR03CTouHB-Ti3kOthBn42aY1q5tNtxhWhSjj8LN8kSqOjqCVygrqNrxOi0.

42 "Constitution of the World Health Organization," *Basic Documents* 45th ed., October 2006, https://www.who.int/governance/eb/who_constitution_en.pdf.

43 World Health Organization Regional Office for Europe, "Health Promotion: A Discussion Document on the Concept and Principles," (Summary Report, *Working Group on Concept and Principles of Health Promotion*, Copenhagen, July 1984), https://apps.who.int/iris/handle/10665/107835.

44 Edwin Choi and Juhan Sonin, "Determinants of Health," *GoInvo*, accessed March 15, 2020, https://www.goinvo.com/vision/determinants-of-health/.

45 Rebecca M. Puhl and Chelsea A. Heuer, "The Stigma of Obesity: A Review and Update," *Obesity* 17, no. 5 (2009): 941–64.

46 Gary D. Foster et al., "Primary Care Physicians' Attitudes About Obesity and Its Treatment," *Obesity Research* 11, no. 10 (2003): 1168–77.

47 Rebecca M. Puhl, Christopher Wharton, and Chelsea Heuer, "Weight Bias Among Dietetics Students: Implications for Treatment Practices," *Journal of the American Dietetic Association* 109, no. 3 (2009): 438–44.

48 William S. Pearson et al., "The Impact of Obesity on Time Spent with the Provider and Number of Medications Managed During Office-Based Physician Visits Using a Cross-Sectional, National Health Survey," *BMC Public Health* 9 (2009): 436.

49 "Ellen Maud Bennett Obituary," *Times Colonist*, published July 14–16, 2018, https://www.legacy.com/obituaries/timescolonist/obituary.aspx?n=ellen-maud-bennett&pid=189588876.

50 Rebecca M. Puhl and Chelsea A. Heuer, "The Stigma of Obesity: A Review and Update," *Obesity* 17, no. 5 (2009): 941–64.

51 Christine Aramburu Alegria Drury and Margaret Louis, "Exploring the Association Between Body Weight, Stigma of Obesity, and Health Care Avoidance," *Journal of the American Academy of Nurse Practitioners* 14, no. 12 (2002): 554–61.

52 Janet Tomiyama et al., "How and Why Weight Stigma Drives the Obesity 'Epidemic' and Harms Health," *BMC Medicine* 16, no. 1 (2018): 123.

53 Brendan Meyer, "At 112, America's Oldest Man Has the Secret to a Long Life: 'Just Keep Living. Don't Die'," *Dallas Morning News*, May 10, 2018, https://www.dallasnews.com/news/healthy-living/2018/05/10/at-112-america-s-oldest-man-has-the-secret-to-a-long-life-just-keep-living-don-t-die/.

54 Dan Buettner, *The Blue Zones: 9 Lessons for Living Longer From the People Who've Lived the Longest*, 2nd ed. (Washington: National Geographic, 2012).

55 Shuangmiao Wang et al., "Contemporary Chinese Centenarians: Health Profiles, Social Support and Relationships in Suixi County," *Archives of Gerontology and Geriatrics* 86 (2020): 103965.

56 Robyn L. Richmond, Jenaleen Law, and Frances Kay-Lambkin, "Physical, Mental, and Cognitive Function in a Convenience Sample of Centenarians in Australia," *Journal of the American Geriatrics Society* 59, no. 6 (2011): 1080–6.

57 Longjian Liu and Craig J. Newschaffer, "Impact of Social Connections on Risk of Heart Disease, Cancer, and All-Cause Mortality among Elderly Americans: Findings from the Second Longitudinal Study of Aging (LSOA II)," *Archives of Gerontology and Geriatrics* 53, no. 2 (2011): 168–73.

58 Dennis Grevenstein et al., "Better Family Relationships— Higher Well-Being: The Connection between Relationship Quality and Health Related Resources," *Mental Health & Prevention* 14 (2019): 200160.

59 "Sleep Deprivation and Deficiency," National Heart, Lung, and Blood Institute (NHLBI), accessed March 16, 2020, https://www.nhlbi.nih.gov/health-topics/sleep-deprivation-and-deficiency.

60 P. Rozin et al., "Attitudes to Food and the Role of Food in Life in the U.S.A., Japan, Flemish Belgium and France: Possible Implications for the Diet–Health Debate," *Appetite* 33, no. 2 (1999): 163–80.

61 Steven N. Blair, "Physical Fitness and All-Cause Mortality: A Prospective Study of Healthy Men and Women," *Journal of the American Medical Association* 262, no. 17 (1989): 2395–401.

62 *Ibid.*

63 Louise Foxcroft, *Calories and Corsets: A History of Dieting Over 2,000 Years* (London: Profile Books, 2013).

64 *Ibid.*

65 Isabel Fletcher, "Defining an Epidemic: the Body Mass Index in British and US Obesity Research 1960–2000," *Sociology of Health & Illness* 36, no. 3 (2013): 338–53.

66 John D. Sorkin, "BMI, Age, and Mortality: The Slaying of a Beautiful Hypothesis by an Ugly Fact," *American Journal of Clinical Nutrition* 99, no. 4 (2014): 759–60.

67 Your Fat Friend, "The Bizarre and Racist History of the BMI," Elemental, published October 15, 2019, https://elemental.medium.com/the-bizarre-and-racist-history-of-the-bmi-7d8dc2aa33bb.

68 The Endocrine Society, "Widely Used Body Fat Measurements Overestimate Fatness In African-Americans, Study Finds," *ScienceDaily*, published June 22, 2009, www.sciencedaily.com/releases/2009/06/090611142407.htm.

69 Susan B. Racette, Susan S. Deusinger, and Robert H. Deusinger, "Obesity: Overview of Prevalence, Etiology, and Treatment," *Physical Therapy* 83, no. 3 (2003): 276–88.

70 S. A. Porter et al., "Abdominal Subcutaneous Adipose Tissue: A Protective Fat Depot?" *Diabetes Care* 32, no. 6 (2009): 1068–75.

71 Linda Bacon, *Health at Every Size: The Surprising Truth About Your Weight*, 2nd ed. (Dallas, TX, BenBella Books, 2010).

72 C. L. Ogden et al., "Mean Body Weight, Height, and Body Mass Index, United States 1960–2002," *Advance Data from Vital and Health Statistics* 347 (2004): 1–17.

73 Katherine M. Flegal et al., "Trends in Obesity Among Adults in the United States, 2005 to 2014," *Journal of the American Medical Association* 315, no. 21 (2016): 2284–91.

74 Charlotte Biltekoff, "The Terror Within: Obesity in Post 9/11 U.S. Life," *American Studies* 48, no. 3 (2007): 29–48.

75 *Ibid.*

76 Ali H. Mokdad et al., "Actual Causes of Death in the United States, 2000," *Journal of the American Medical Association* 291, no. 10 (2004): 1238–45.

77 Katherine M. Flegal et al., "Excess Deaths Associated With Underweight, Overweight, and Obesity," *Journal of the American Medical Association* 293, no. 15 (2005): 1861–7.

78 Andrew Pollack, "A.M.A. Recognizes Obesity as a Disease," *New York Times*, June 18, 2013, https://www.nytimes.com/2013/06/19/business/ama-recognizes-obesity-as-a-disease.html.

79 "The U.S. Weight Loss and Diet Control Market," *Research and Markets*, published February 2019, https://www.researchandmarkets.com/research/qm2gts/the_72_billion?w=4.

80 Tomohide Yamada et al., "Male Pattern Baldness and Its Association with Coronary Heart Disease: A Meta-Analysis," *BMJ Open* 3, no. 4 (2013).

81 Kelley Strohacker and Brian K. Mcfarlin, "Influence of Obesity Physical Inactivity and Weight Cycling on Chronic Inflammation," *Frontiers in Bioscience* E2, no. 1 (2010): 98–104.

82 Janet Tomiyama et al., "Low Calorie Dieting Increases Cortisol," *Psychosomatic Medicine* 72, no. 4 (2010): 357–64.

83 J-P Montani et al., "Weight Cycling During Growth and Beyond as a Risk Factor for Later Cardiovascular Diseases: The 'Repeated Overshoot' Theory," *International Journal of Obesity* 30, no. S4 (2006): S58–66; erratum-ibid., *International Journal of Obesity* 34, no. 7 (2010): 1230.

84 Vanessa A. Diaz, Arch G. Mainous, and Charles J. Everett, "The Association Between Weight Fluctuation And Mortality: Results From A Population-Based Cohort Study," *Journal of Community Health* 30, no. 3 (2005): 153–65.

85 Gregory Pavela et al., "Socioeconomic Status, Risk of Obesity, and the Importance of Albert J. Stunkard," *Current Obesity Reports* 5, no. 1 (2016): 132–9.

86 Jens Ludwig et al., "Neighborhoods, Obesity, and Diabetes: A Randomized Social Experiment," *New England Journal of Medicine* 365, no. 16 (2011): 1509–19.

87 Daniel L. McGee, "Body Mass Index and Mortality: A Meta-Analysis Based on Person-Level Data from Twenty-Six Observational Studies," *Annals of Epidemiology* 15, no. 2 (2005): 87–97.

88 Janet Tomiyama et al., "Misclassification of Cardiometabolic Health When Using Body Mass Index Categories in NHANES 2005–2012," *International Journal of Obesity* 40, no. 5 (2016): 883–6.

89 Christy Harrison, *Anti-Diet: Reclaim Your Time, Money, Well-Being and Happiness Through Intuitive Eating* (New York: Hachette Book Group, 2019).

90 Ellyn Satter, "Hierarchy of Food Needs," *Journal of Nutrition Education and Behavior* 39, no. 5 (2007): S187–8.

91 Jordan Skrynka and Benjamin T. Vincent, "Hunger Increases Delay Discounting of Food and Non-Food Rewards," *Psychonomic Bulletin & Review* 26, no. 5 (2019): 1729–37.

92 Jennifer L. Gaudiani, *Sick Enough: A Guide to the Medical Complications of Eating Disorders* (New York: Routledge, 2019).

93 Miguel Toribio-Mateas, "Harnessing the Power of Microbiome Assessment Tools as Part of Neuroprotective Nutrition and Lifestyle Medicine Interventions," *Microorganisms* 6, no. 2 (2018): 35.

94 Seema Gulati, Anoop Misra, and Ravindra M Pandey, "Effects of 3 g of Soluble Fiber from Oats on Lipid Levels of Asian Indians—A Randomized Controlled, Parallel Arm Study," *Lipids in Health and Disease* 16, no. 1 (2017): 71.

95 Roy M. Pitkin, "Folate and Neural Tube Defects," *American Journal of Clinical Nutrition* 85, no. 1 (2007): 285S–8S.

96 Ab Latif Wani, Sajad Ahmad Bhat, and Anjum Ara, "Omega-3 Fatty Acids and the Treatment of Depression: A Review of Scientific Evidence," *Integrative Medicine Research* 4, no. 3 (2015): 132–41.

97 Peter Soumia, Chopra Sandeep, and Jacob Jubbin, "A Fish a Day, Keeps the Cardiologist Away!—A Review of the Effect of Omega-3 Fatty Acids in the Cardiovascular System," *Indian Journal of Endocrinology and Metabolism* 17, no. 3 (2013): 422–9.

98 L. Schwingshackl et al., "Olive Oil in the Prevention and Management of Type 2 Diabetes Mellitus: A Systematic Review and Meta-Analysis of Cohort Studies and Intervention Trials," *Nutrition & Diabetes* 7, no. 4 (2017): e262.

99 Dagfinn Aune et al., "Fruit and Vegetable Intake and the Risk of Cardiovascular Disease, Total Cancer and All-Cause Mortality—A Systematic Review and Dose-Response Meta-Analysis of Prospective Studies," *International Journal of Epidemiology* 46, no. 3 (2017): 1029–56.

100 Carl K. Winter and Josh M. Katz, "Dietary Exposure to Pesticide Residues from Commodities Alleged to Contain the Highest Contamination Levels," *Journal of Toxicology* (2011): 1–7.

101 Robert Krieger, *Perspective on Pesticide Residues in Fruits and Vegetables* (Riverside: University of California-Riverside, n.d.), https://www.safefruitsandveggies.com/wp-content/uploads/2019/02/pesticides-in-perspective.pdf.

102 Dagfinn Aune et al., "Whole Grain Consumption and Risk of Cardiovascular Disease, Cancer, and All Cause and Cause Specific Mortality: Systematic Review and Dose-Response Meta-Analysis of Prospective Studies," *BMJ* 353 (2016): i2716.

103 Leonora N. Panlasigui and Lilian U. Thompson, "Blood Glucose Lowering Effects of Brown Rice in Normal and Diabetic Subjects," *International Journal of Food Sciences and Nutrition* 57, no. 3–4 (2006): 151–8.

104 James J. Dinicolantonio and James H O'Keefe, "Effects of Dietary Fats on Blood Lipids: A Review of Direct Comparison Trials," *Open Heart* 5, no. 2 (2018): e000871.

105 P. E. Miller, M. Van Elswyk, and D. D. Alexander, "Long-Chain Omega-3 Fatty Acids Eicosapentaenoic Acid and Docosahexaenoic Acid and Blood Pressure: A Meta-Analysis of Randomized Controlled Trials," *American Journal of Hypertension* 27, no. 7 (2014): 88596.

106 Philip C. Calder, "Omega-3 Fatty Acids and Inflammatory Processes: from Molecules to Man," *Biochemical Society Transactions* 45, no. 5 (2017): 1105–15.

107 Liana C. Del Gobbo et al., "Ω-3 Polyunsaturated Fatty Acid Biomarkers and Coronary Heart Disease: Pooling Project of 19 Cohort Studies," *JAMA Internal Medicine* 176, no.8 (2016): 1155–66.

108 William Raphael and Lorraine Sordillo, "Dietary Polyunsaturated Fatty Acids and Inflammation: The Role of Phospholipid Biosynthesis," *International Journal of Molecular Sciences* 14, no. 10 (2013): 21167–88.

109 Dong D. Wang et al., "Association of Specific Dietary Fats With Total and Cause-Specific Mortality," *JAMA Internal Medicine* 176, no. 8 (2016): 1134–45.

110 Russell J. De Souza et al., "Intake of Saturated and Trans Unsaturated Fatty Acids and Risk of All Cause Mortality, Cardiovascular Disease, and Type 2 Diabetes: Systematic Review and Meta-Analysis of Observational Studies," *BMJ* (2015): 351.

111 "Traditional Diets," Oldways, accessed March 16, 2020, https://oldwayspt.org/traditional-diets.

112 Emma J. Derbyshire, "Flexitarian Diets and Health: A Review of the Evidence-Based Literature," *Frontiers in Nutrition* 3 (2016): 55.

113 D. F. Hebeisen et al., "Increased Concentrations of Omega-3 Fatty Acids in Milk and Platelet Rich Plasma of Grass-Fed Cows," *International Journal for Vitamin and Nutrition Research* 63, no. 3 (1993): 229–33.

114 T. R. Dhiman et al., "Conjugated Linoleic Acid Content of Milk from Cows Fed Different Diets," *Journal of Dairy Science* 82, no. 10 (1999): 2146–56.

115 D. Baran et al., "Dietary Modification with Dairy Products for Preventing Vertebral Bone Loss in Premenopausal Women: A Three-Year Prospective Study," *Journal of Clinical Endocrinology & Metabolism* 70, no. 1 (1990): 264–70.

116 P. C. Elwood et al., "Milk Drinking, Ischaemic Heart Disease and Ischaemic Stroke II. Evidence from Cohort Studies," *European Journal of Clinical Nutrition* 58, no. 5 (2004): 718–24.

117 Alessandra Bordoni et al., "Dairy Products and Inflammation: A Review of the Clinical Evidence," *Critical Reviews in Food Science and Nutrition* 57, no. 12 (2017): 2497–525.

118 Heather Hall et al., "Glucotypes Reveal New Patterns of Glucose Dysregulation," *PLOS Biology* 16, no. 7 (2018): e2005143.

119 Yuren Wang et al., "Plasma Asprosin Concentrations Are Increased in Individuals with Glucose Dysregulation and Correlated with Insulin Resistance and First-Phase Insulin Secretion," *Mediators of Inflammation* 2018: 1–7.

120 Ashley E. Mason et al., "Effects of a Mindfulness-Based Intervention on Mindful Eating, Sweets Consumption, and Fasting Glucose Levels in Obese Adults: Data from the SHINE Randomized Controlled Trial," *Journal of Behavioral Medicine* 39, no. 2 (2015): 201–13.

121 F. S. Atkinson, K. Foster-Powell, and J. C. Brand-Miller, "International Tables of Glycemic Index and Glycemic Load Values: 2008," *Diabetes Care* 31, no. 12 (2008): 2281–3.

122 Silvano Gallus et al., "Artificial Sweeteners and Cancer Risk in a Network of Case–Control Studies," *Annals of Oncology* 18, no. 1 (2007): 40–4.

123 H. E. Ford et al., "Effects of Oral Ingestion of Sucralose on Gut Hormone Response and Appetite in Healthy Normal-Weight Subjects," *European Journal of Clinical Nutrition* 65, no. 4 (2011): 508–13.

124 *Ibid.*

125 Stephen D. Anton et al., "Effects of Stevia, Aspartame, and Sucrose on Food Intake, Satiety, and Postprandial Glucose and Insulin Levels," *Appetite* 55, no. 1 (2010): 37–43.

126 L. Hallberg et al., "Iron Absorption from Southeast Asian Diets. II. Role of Various Factors That Might Explain Low Absorption," *American Journal of Clinical Nutrition* 30, no. 4 (1977): 539–48.

127 Michelle E. Watts, Roger Pocock, and Charles Claudianos, "Brain Energy and Oxygen Metabolism: Emerging Role in Normal Function and Disease," *Frontiers in Molecular Neuroscience* 11 (2018): 216.

128 B. J. Fogg, *Tiny Habits: The Small Changes That Change Everything* (Boston: Houghton Mifflin Harcourt, 2019).

129 Gaby Judah, Benjamin Gardner, and Robert Aunger, "Forming a Flossing Habit: An Exploratory Study of the Psychological Determinants of Habit Formation," *British Journal of Health Psychology* 18, no. 2 (2012): 338–53.

130 Peter M. Gollwitzer and Paschal Sheeran, "Implementation Intentions and Goal Achievement: A Meta Analysis of Effects and Processes," *Advances in Experimental Social Psychology* 38 (2006): 69–119.

131 Sarah Milne, Sheina Orbell, and Paschal Sheeran, "Combining Motivational and Volitional Interventions to Promote Exercise Participation: Protection Motivation Theory and Implementation Intentions," *British Journal of Health Psychology* 7, no. 2 (2002): 163–84.

132 "The Broaden-and-Build Theory of Positive Emotions," *Philosophical Transactions of the Royal Society* B 359 (2004): 1367–77.

133 Patty Van Cappellen et al., "Positive Affective Processes Underlie Positive Health Behaviour Change," *Psychology & Health* 33, no. 1 (2017): 77–97.

134 Barbara L. Fredrickson, "Positive Emotions Broaden and Build," *Advances in Experimental Social Psychology* 47 (2013): 1–53.

135 Barbara L. Fredrickson, "The Broaden-and-Build Theory of Positive Emotions," *Philosophical Transactions of the Royal Society* B 359 (2004): 1367–77.

136 F. M. Sirois, R. Kitner, and J. K. Hirsch, "Self-Compassion, Affect, and Health-Promoting Behaviors," *Health Psychology* 34, no. 6 (2015): 661–9.

137 Dirk Jan Stenvers et al., "Nutrition and the Circadian Timing System," Progress in Brain Research *The Neurobiology of Circadian Timing* 199 (2012): 359–76.

138 Kazue Okamoto-Mizuno and Koh Mizuno, "Effects of Thermal Environment on Sleep and Circadian Rhythm," *Journal of Physiological Anthropology* 31, no. 14 (2012): 1–9.

139 Mariana G. Figueiro et al., "The Impact of Light from Computer Monitors on Melatonin Levels in College Students," *Neuroendocrinology Letters* 32, no. 2 (2011): 158–63.

140 M. Alexandra Kredlow et al., "The Effects of Physical Activity on Sleep: A Meta-Analytic Review," *Journal of Behavioral Medicine* 38, no. 3 (2015): 427–49.

141 Jonathan Halpern et al., "Yoga for Improving Sleep Quality and Quality of Life for Older Adults," *Alternative Therapies in Health and Medicine* 20, no. 3 (2014): 37–46.

142 Irshaad O. Ebrahim et al., "Alcohol and Sleep I: Effects on Normal Sleep," *Alcoholism: Clinical and Experimental Research* 37, no. 4 (2013): 539–49.

143 Yogesh Singh, Ratna Sharma, and Anjana Talwar, "Immediate and Long-Term Effects of Meditation on Acute Stress Reactivity, Cognitive Functions, and Intelligence," *Alternative Therapies* 18, no. 6 (2012): 46–53.

144 Nicole L. Glazer et al., "Sustained and Shorter Bouts of Physical Activity Are Related to Cardiovascular Health," *Medicine & Science in Sports & Exercise* 45, no. 1 (2013): 109–15.

145 Harriet Frost, "How to Start Building Positive Body Image with Ashlee Bennett," September 20, 2019, in *Don't Salt My Game*, produced by Laura Thomas, podcast, MP3 audio, 64:43, http://www.laurathomasphd.co.uk/podcast/ep-ashlee-bennett/.

146 Bryony Bamford and Emma Halliwell, "Investigating the Role of Attachment in Social Comparison Theories of Eating Disorders within a Non-Clinical Female Population," *European Eating Disorders Review* 17, no. 5 (2009): 371–9.

147 Janet Polivy, "What's That You're Eating? Social Comparison and Eating Behavior," *Journal of Eating Disorders* 5 (2017): 18.

148 Barbara Vad Andersen and Grethe Hyldig, "Consumers' View on Determinants to Food Satisfaction. A Qualitative Approach," *Appetite* 95 (2015): 9–16.

149 E. Jéquier, "Carbohydrates as a Source of Energy," *American Journal of Clinical Nutrition* 59, no. 3 (1994): 682S–5S.

150 "Appendix 7: Nutritional Goals for Age-Sex Groups Based on Dietary Reference Intakes and Dietary Guidelines Recommendations," *Dietary Guidelines for Americans 2015–2020*, 8th ed., December 2015, https://health.gov/our-work/food-nutrition/2015-2020-dietary-guidelines/guidelines/appendix-7/.

151 Yeong Yeh Lee, Askin Erdogan, and Satish S C Rao, "How to Assess Regional and Whole Gut Transit Time with Wireless Motility Capsule," *Journal of Neurogastroenterology and Motility* 20, no. 2 (2014): 265–70.

152 Elizabeth A. Pletsch and Bruce R. Hamaker, "Brown Rice Compared to White Rice Slows Gastric Emptying in Humans," *European Journal of Clinical Nutrition* 72, no. 3 (2018): 367–73.

153 Rachel L. Batterham et al., "Critical Role for Peptide YY in Protein-Mediated Satiation and Body-Weight Regulation," *Cell Metabolism* 4, no. 3 (2006): 223–33.

154 Wendy A. M. Blom et al., "Effect of a High-Protein Breakfast on the Postprandial Ghrelin Response," *American Journal of Clinical Nutrition* 83, no. 2 (2006): 211–20.

155 Adam Drewnowski and Eva Almiron-Roig, "Human Perceptions and Preferences for Fat-Rich Foods," in *Fat Detection: Taste, Texture, and Post Ingestive Effects*, eds. Jean-Pierre Montmayeur and Johannes le Coutre (Boca Raton: CRC Press, 2010).

156 Adam Drewnowski, "Why Do We Like Fat?," *Journal of the American Dietetic Association* 97, no. 7 (1997): S58–S62.

157 P. Rozin et al., "Attitudes to Food and the Role of Food in Life in the U.S.A., Japan, Flemish Belgium and France: Possible Implications for the Diet–Health Debate," *Appetite* 33, no. 2 (1999): 163–80.

158 *Ibid.*

159 Linshan Li et al., "Selected Nutrient Analyses of Fresh, Fresh-Stored, and Frozen Fruits and Vegetables," *Journal of Food Composition and Analysis* 59 (2017): 8–17.

Index